Integrative Acupressure

A Hands-On Guide
to Balancing the Body's Structure and
Energy for Health and Healing

Sam McClellan

with Tom Monte

A Perigee Book

A Perigee Book
Published by The Berkley Publishing Group
A member of Penguin Putnam Inc.
375 Hudson Street
New York, New York 10014

First edition: December 1998

Published simultaneously in Canada.

The Penguin Putnam Inc. World Wide Web site address is
http://www.penguinputnam.com

Library of Congress Cataloging-in-Publication Data

McClellan, Sam.
    Integrative acupressure : a hands-on guide to balancing the body's
structure and energy for health and healing / Sam McClellan, with
Tom Monte.—1st ed.
        p.   cm.
    "A Perigee book."
    ISBN 0-399-52441-X (tp)
    1. Acupressure.   2. Acupuncture points.   3. Self-care, Health.
4. Exercise therapy.   I. Monte, Tom.   II. Title.
RM723.A27M34   1998
615.8'22—dc21   98-3034
                                                            CIP

Printed in the United States of America

10   9   8   7   6   5   4   3   2   1

CONTENTS

Introduction

By the time we reach adult-
hood, most of us live in bodies that are riddled with odd physical
distortions. If you were to look at your body in a mirror, you
might conclude that you've been reshaped over the years by a
powerful force with a quirky sense of humor. These distortions
seem to turn up in every possible location. Most of us, for example, have a shoulder or hip that is higher than its respective
counterpart. Some people have hips that are not directly in line
with their chests. Either the hips are set back slightly so that they
appear to be chasing after the chest as a person walks down the
street, or they're a little forward of the chest, thus leading the
way. Take a look at people's profiles and you'll notice that their
heads are usually well forward of the shoulders—the old vulture
look. And if we lie down with our legs stretched to their maximum, many of us will find that one leg is longer than the other.
Eighty percent of American adults—more than 150 million people—suffer from back pain that is a direct result of misalignment
of the spine and vertebrae. But if you work on people's backs,
as I do, you'll realize that by the time people reach thirty-five or
forty, not only are the vertebrae misaligned, but most of us have
rib cages that are bulged on the left or the right sides, as if the
organs beneath the bones were ballooned and misshapen.

In fact, such imbalances are the norm for most of us. It is the
rare person who doesn't have a set of pronounced physical distortions. At first these misalignments appear to us as startling,
even shocking. But upon closer examination you will discover
that your body is in fact a chain of distortions, each one compensating for the next. Even the grossest misalignment is just the

tip of the iceberg. What appears as a strange and even funny imbalance—one leg longer than the other, for example—corresponds to equally profound imbalances in our muscles, organs, and even our cells.

Two questions jump out at us: What do these imbalances mean, and how can I correct them?

The answer to both of these questions lies in the practice of acupressure. Acupressure can decode the language of the body and thereby reveal the inner you. It is also the tool—or set of tools—that can correct imbalances and restore your health. When I say health, I mean freedom from the acute and restricting symptoms of illness. I also mean an awakening to your truest and deepest self. The ultimate purpose of acupressure is to help people overcome sickness and disability and become whole. Being whole is essential to the discovery of your unique self, which is to say, the person you came into the world to be.

In the strictest sense, acupressure is a method of using finger and hand pressure on specific points on the body to improve health. It is based on the ancient practice of acupuncture, which uses needles to stimulate electromagnetic energy that flows along specific pathways within the body. That energy is known as the life force or, in Chinese medicine, as Qi (pronounced "chee"). It flows along pathways, known as meridians, to every organ, system, and cell. By boosting or balancing the energy, or life force, flowing to organs and tissues, the therapist can initiate healing. Acupressure applies these same principles, but instead of using needles to cause healing, the acupressurist uses finger and hand pressure to stimulate points along the meridians. By pressing these points, an acupressurist stimulates life force to flow along the meridian, or pathway of energy, to a specific organ or part of the body, thereby triggering the healing process.

As a practitioner of acupressure for more than two decades, I have taken the practice beyond its traditional limits to combine energetic work with structural alignment. I call this practice Integrative Acupressure. Like traditional acupuncture and acupressure, Integrative Acupressure is based on Chinese medicine. I manipulate the body's life force, or Qi, to promote physical, psychological, and spiritual healing. But many of the problems that have presented themselves in my practice have required that I go beyond working strictly on meridians and energy imbalances to work also on releasing muscle tension and correcting structural misalignment. Therefore, Integrative Acupressure also draws upon the fundamentals of anatomy and physiology, physical therapy, and therapeutic massage. What makes such a synthesis of disciplines possible is its basis in the all-encompassing system of Chinese medicine. As you will see in this book, Chinese medicine is that rare paradox of being broad and all-embracing, and at the same time specific and direct.

In the pages that follow, I will provide a complete course in Integrative Acupressure—everything from boosting Qi flow along specific meridians and organs to correcting muscular and structural imbalances. For those looking for answers to personal issues—and I hope this includes every reader, regardless of his or her professional direction—this book will help you understand yourself in a whole new light. I also provide many self-help methods, such as key points to massage and foot reflexology, that can greatly improve your own health and vitality. The self-help tools that I offer will address both short- and long-term issues. You can stimulate these points yourself to relieve symptoms and to heal underlying imbalances that may be causing one or another disorder.

There is more to this practice, however, than pressing points, balancing tension, and correcting misalignments. Before you can begin to correct imbalances in yourself or another person, you must be able to assess where the imbalances lie and what the most likely weaknesses are. To that end, this book presents a comprehensive explanation of traditional Chinese diagnostic techniques including using the concepts of yin and yang and the Five Element theory.

For those who wish to become professional acupressure practitioners, this book will provide you with the foundation for a career in one of the most powerful healing arts. Whatever your reasons for coming to acupressure, this practice requires you to develop understanding and compassion for those whom you wish to assist, including yourself. Like many traditional healing practices, acupressure makes its greatest demands on each of us to grow as human beings, and thus to better understand life.

The Body as Structure and Energy

We can think of the human body in many ways, but a revealing metaphor is to see it architecturally, as a living work of art that has design and structure, or like a building. If we look at the body as an architect would, we can see how all the parts relate to each other; how the whole is created by the relationship among the parts; and how those parts add up to more than their sum. In other words, there is more to us than this constellation of individual bones, organs, systems, and senses.

Like all buildings, the body has a superstructure. Instead of steel girders, ours is a skeleton composed of 206 bones. The superstructure is supported and moved by an array of tendons, muscles, and ligaments that connect the bones and move them individually and collectively. Supported within this structural framework and its muscular system are the organs, nervous system, blood vessels, blood, and lymph system. Each part is wrapped in thin, strong fascial membranes, and the whole building is wrapped in skin.

When we consider the relationship between the superstructure—that is, the bones—and the organs, we begin to see how much the organs depend on the integrity of the structure. Change just one aspect of the structure—say, the rib cage—and you affect the entire organism. The ribs and diaphragm muscles make breathing possible. If the ribs are injured or prevented from expanding and contracting optimally, your breathing can be severely restricted. That, in turn, limits your capacity to take in oxygen, which reduces your energy. Restricted breathing also prevents the elimination of carbon dioxide, causing waste products to build up within the system. As waste accumulates, the immune system is worked endlessly, until it is weakened and eventually compromised. Since the blood and lymph now contain more waste products, all the organs—especially the blood-cleansing organs—are burdened by the accumulation of toxins. The result is a greater susceptibility to infections, colds, and ultimately more serious illnesses. Elderly adults experience a seemingly endless array of health problems that result from structural changes alone. By changing one simple part of the body's structure the entire health and future of the person will be affected.

The opposite is also true: Changes in organs affect skeletal structure, such as when an organ swells or becomes overly contracted. By becoming swollen and hard, the liver can cause the rib cage to bulge and the right shoulder to rise. By becoming contracted and hardened, the left lung can cause the chest to shrink and the right shoulder to drop. By expanding and becoming swollen, the stomach and small intestines can pull on the spine, forcing vertebrae to contract upon one another and pinch nerves. The result can be chronic back pain.

Structural integrity, of both the skeleton and the organs, is vital to our overall health and well-being. But we are more than structure. Another factor—an even more fundamental one—plays an essential role in our health.

STRUCTURE AND ENERGY: COMPLEMENTARY OPPOSITES

I mentioned earlier that well-worn aphorism that the body is more than the sum of its parts. That "more" is energy. Our physical structures would decay rather rapidly if it were not for the presence of energy. Deprived of energy, all the bones, muscles, organs, and tissues would decay, and thus return to their origin, the earth. To put it another way: Without energy, structure collapses.

From a Chinese medical point of view, the body is a beautiful balance between kinetic and potential energy. Kinetic energy is movement and expression; potential energy is matter and mass. In health, potential energy is continually being turned into kinetic energy, or the energy of movement. Yet there must be a balance between these two. Excess potential energy leads to stagnation and illnesses of accumulation, such as obesity, atherosclerosis and other cardiovascular diseases, kidney stones, intestinal polyps, and cancers. Too much kinetic energy leads to excessive weight loss and illnesses that are characterized by deficiency, such as anemia (low hemoglobin), hypoglycemia (low blood sugar), osteoporosis (porous bones), and poor nutrient absorption and assimilation, just to name a few.

Our bodies are always trying to balance these opposites—kinetic and potential energy, motion and structure, utilization and storage—to maintain health.

Conceptually, we can think about energy as an abstract thing, but in daily life, and especially when it comes to the physical body, energy and structure are inextricably joined as complementary opposites.

They greatly influence one another. Take tension, for example. Remember the last time you were behind on a deadline and racing to catch up? Go back to that period and reexperience it for a moment: Your mind is going in ten different directions at once. That mental energy is being converted into shortness of breath and muscular tension, which you may be holding in your pelvis, lower back, stomach, shoulders, and neck. As we will see later on, the locations where each of us stores tension are well established. The most obvious place you experience such tension is your shoulders: the clavicle, scapula, and upper rib bones are pulled tight by your shoulder muscles. But muscles elsewhere in your body are equally affected, although you may not be conscious of the tension in those places.

All of these contracted muscles will pull bones, ligaments, and tendons and thus cause structural changes. If the tension is chronic, as it is for most of us living in the modern world, the integrity of the body is eventually changed. These changes are gradual—so gradual, in fact, that we aren't aware of them until that fateful day when our backs give out and we're laid up for a few days or a few weeks with unbelievable back pain.

Tension changes structure, which is a short and simple way of saying that your mind shapes your body. When you were a child, you were relaxed and open while you played, ate, slept, or wet your diaper. However, whenever you did something that your parents didn't want you to do, you probably were scolded by them. Your body's immediate reaction was to recoil from the powerful emotions of your parents. That recoiling creates muscle tension that must ultimately be released if the body is to return to its supple and healthy condition.

For many children, scolding—and even physical abuse—occurs routinely, causing chronic patterns of psychological and physical tension they may never learn to release. Such patterns of tension become well entrenched in the muscles, tendons, and ligaments and affect growth and behavioral patterns. (I'll discuss such patterns, and what can be done about them, later on in this book.) The opportunities to be traumatized as a child seem endless. All of us were frightened, shocked, saddened, and angered as children, and each of these events created tension within our bodies.

Tension prevents blood, lymph, and Qi from flowing to these areas. Each area becomes cool, stagnant, and numb. Feeling is reduced in that part of the body. By diminishing our ability to feel and experience life with that part of our bodies, we are in effect separating the mind from the body.

As adults, job or family difficulties create ongoing and sometimes chronic stresses, which are translated into physical and psychological tension. When left unresolved and unreleased, such tension gradually diminishes the flow of blood, oxygen, and lymph. The tension prevents toxins from flowing from the affected area. Finally, it diminishes the flow of electromagnetic energy to that part of the body, so that you begin to lack the biological and electrical resources necessary for health.

In addition to tension, injury and trauma can also affect structure and create long-term physical problems. A car accident or a blow during a football game can remain chronically inflamed for years. A sickness or fever can affect specific parts of the body long after the acute symptoms have faded. An injured knee or other joint can result in inflammation that remains intractable. The lymph and bursae (the fluid-filled sacs within the joints) can remain inflamed, indicating that the area has never fully healed.

We are witness to the essential truth that the body contains the past, present, and future. When we look at the body, we see the past in the form of imbalances created by a person's life experiences, thoughts, and emotions. We see the present in the form of the current condition, which may be inflammation, pain, and blocked blood flow. We see the future in the form of the person's potential to heal and become themselves. The body, mind, and spirit are one.

When the acupressurist begins to work on an imbalance or injury, he or she is reintroducing the person's awareness to a part of the body that has been neglected, sometimes for many, many years. Naturally, memories begin to surface. The tension that is gradually released may stimulate a flood of emotion. Healing takes place: physically, psychologically, and spiritually.

I like to think of this as cellular memory, because as I work on a person, I am not just releasing the tension in that part of the body, but awakening that person to a part of the body that has been near death since the original trauma set in. A specific set of events—memories of which still linger in the unconscious—caused this part of the body to become numb. This tension can be seen as energy that is blocked or trapped within the body. It exists in the form of memories—sometimes powerful and painful memories—and in specific physical locations within the body itself.

The human body is the realm in which all of these mysteries converge and become accessible to us. Therefore, when we work on the body, we are treating the mind and spirit. When we heal an injury, we are reconciling ourselves with the past and allowing our true natures to guide and create our future. This is why I say that healing is not merely the elimination of symptoms, but the emergence of the true you.

THE POWER OF ACUPRESSURE TO HEAL

Scoliosis is lateral curvature of the spine, meaning that the spine curves to the left or right of the midpoint on the back. Just about everyone has some lateral curves in their spines, but the term scoliosis is not applied until there is at least ten degrees of curvature or better. In fact, twenty degrees of curvature is not uncommon. One in every ten people has scoliosis; two in every thousand will need to be monitored and treated; and one in every thousand will need scoliosis surgery. Scoliosis is considered a serious problem when the curve reaches thirty degrees or more because of the effects such a curve has on the person's organs.

The only two treatments recognized by Western medicine are back-bracing and surgery. If the back brace does not improve the condition, the standard protocol is to perform a fusion of several vertebrae of the spine. The fusion surgery usually corrects the curve by more than half, but in the process leaves the person unable to bend the back in the area of the fusion. Typical fusion surgeries occur from thoracic 3 or 4 (found in the upper part of the body) down to lumbar 3 or 4, a significant part of the back.

The most common form of scoliosis is idiopathic scoliosis, literally meaning curvature of unknown origin. This form constitutes 80 percent of the scoliosis cases diagnosed every year, and the vast majority of these are adolescent and preadolescent girls.

Over the years, I have worked with numerous children with significant scoliosis ranging from mild to severe. In all but the most extreme cases, I was able to reverse the scoliotic curve, usually to a fraction of its initial deviation. In what is so far our best-documented case, involving a fifteen-year-old girl, I was able to bring a twenty-three-degree curve down to eleven degrees in just eight weeks. When the family went to their physician for an X ray, the doctor put the most recent film up on the lighted view box and said, "It's eleven degrees. There must have been a mistake in the original diagnosis."

"There were numerous diagnoses," the father said. "Could all of them have been wrong?"

When the doctor insisted that they were in error, a heated discussion followed, especially between the girl's mother and the doctor. For forty-five minutes, the doctor insisted that nothing could reverse scoliosis. Therefore, all previous diagnoses must have been mistakes.

I continue to see the young girl for treatments and her back has remained in good health, without a return to the serious curvature she once had.

While there are many techniques used to balance relatively extreme sco-liosis, I used two steps in restoring this particular spine.

The first thing to realize is that the spine is curved because the muscles that keep the vertebrae aligned are in spasm, meaning the muscles are pull-ing the vertebrae left and right with unequal pressure locked in contraction. This causes the spine to curve. Therefore, the practitioner's first step is to get the muscles to relax, or release. Once the muscles regain their full range of motion—meaning that they can contract and expand more fluidly—they will reassume their normal or "healthy" relaxed state.

Within the body is a programmed state of balance or health. In the case of the spine, that means once the muscles are restored to health, they will natu-rally apply the appropriate tension to the vertebrae so that the spine's integ-rity and alignment is restored. Therefore, the first step a practitioner must take is to get the muscles out of spasm. For this client, I did it by gently knead-ing the muscles to break up and release the tension. At the same time, I real-ized that the acupressure points that provided Qi to the muscles and vertebrae—those close to the spine as well as at other points elsewhere on the body—were blocked and knotted, as if they had become bundles of con-gested energy. Thus the second step is to release these points by applying pres-sure directly into the center of the point, and then moving the Qi away from the center. As I will describe later on, this is called release and dispersal.

This process of releasing the muscles and the points effectively took the muscles out of spasm and balanced Qi throughout the back. Week after week, I did this until the alignment of the spine was gradually restored.

THE DANCE OF OPPOSITES

To create healing, we must understand and work with the laws of the body. One of the most fundamental and practical laws is that all movement is made possible through the reaction of opposites.

Artists know this fact very well. Whenever an artist draws a person, say, reaching for a book that rests on a shelf above the person's head, the artist notes the relationship between the hips and the shoulders. When the right shoulder, arm, and hip are raised to reach the book, the left shoulder and hip point downward. Looked at holistically, the body appears to be a series of perfectly balanced opposites—the right side performing one set of ac-tions, while the left balances the body by doing the exact opposite.

All physical movement is made possible through the balancing of oppo-sites. Just walk down the street and notice all the opposites that are harmo-nized as you move: A single step usually consists of the right leg and left arm moving forward together, while the left leg and right arm stay back. Reciprocal motions make the next step possible. Your heartbeat is a perfectly co-ordinated couplet of opposites—systole and diastole. So, too, is your breath.

Opposites are the body's tools, you might say. In health, the body balances opposites to create both motion and harmony. In sickness, it uses opposites to compensate for injuries and weaknesses—both physical and mental—to keep you going. Looked at for the larger picture, opposites will tell a story about the body.

This is why the body, when injured, will attempt to deal with that injury by creating a compensatory imbalance for that injury. Take the spine, for example. Sometimes you will see the lower part of the spine—the lumbar vertebrae and the sacrum—turn slightly to the left. Often, the upper part of the spine will attempt to compensate for this curve by turning to the right, creating an S shape. This compensation, of course, will affect how the neck supports the head and whether the pelvis and hips sit correctly in their joints. Also, the S-shaped curve will cause the spinal vertebrae, disks, and nerves to be squeezed. The result is back and shoulder pain and headaches, problems that affect millions today.

As any engineer, physicist, or chemist will tell you, opposites make energy possible. When we work with opposites, we are working with energy.

HIGHWAYS FOR THE LIFE FORCE

As products of Western culture, we have no developed understanding of how energy travels in the body and no real corollary to the Chinese model of acupuncture meridians. For us, energy is a generalized force that drives material objects, including the body. However, the Chinese have created an intricate system to understand how energy moves within the body, and how it connects the body, mind, and spirit. That system is acupuncture, which is based upon the theory that a universal energy, or life force, infuses all animate and inanimate things. The Chinese maintain that within the human body the life force flows along specific pathways, or meridians, to every organ, system, and cell within the body.

Nonetheless, Western science has been able to demonstrate in its own terms that the human body is, indeed, an electromagnetic unit. In fact, scientists are proving in the laboratory that the human body is animated by a complex web of electrical energy, and that this underlying energy can be enhanced to bring about healing. Among the leaders in this field of research is Robert Becker, M.D., an orthopedic surgeon and professor at the State University of New York (SUNY). Dr. Becker and his colleagues have shown that a variety of techniques can boost the body's underlying electrical currents, which in turn strengthens the body's healing functions, including the immune, endocrine, and nervous systems. Among the techniques Dr. Becker has shown to be effective at strengthening the body's energy system are acupuncture, certain dietary practices, and healing through touch.

In his book *Cross Currents: The Perils of Electropollution, the Promise of Electromedicine* (Jeremy P. Tarcher, 1990), Dr. Becker reported his findings after years of study in the laboratory.

Becker and his colleagues placed sensitive electronic equipment on subjects' bodies and measured whether electromagnetic energy increased during acupuncture and whether it flowed along specific pathways. In *Cross Currents*, he reports: "We found that about 25 percent of the acupuncture points on the human forearm did exist, in that they had specific, reproducible, and significant electrical parameters and could be found in all subjects tested. Next, we looked at the meridians that seemed to connect these points. We found that these meridians had the electrical characteristics of transmission lines, while nonmeridian skin did not."

He and others have shown that by boosting the body's own electrical currents, the immune system and vital organs are also strengthened. Researchers have also demonstrated that the very act of healing is electrical in nature. That is, when the body is injured or ill, it struggles to increase the electrical energy flowing to the site of the injury or illness. This research forms the basis of a potentially revolutionary form of health care that scientists are calling electromedicine. It has the potential to link modern science with ancient healing practices to create a truly unified medical system.

Of course, the Chinese do not regard these channels of energy as electrical, but as a larger life force that infuses and animates the body. That life force, or Qi, is the living energy behind biochemistry. When the life force leaves the body at the time of death, the body—and all its chemical reactions—is revealed for what it is: a matrix of earthly substances that quickly decay.

As long as the life force infuses the body optimally—including every organ, system, and sense—the body enjoys good health and vitality. When the life force becomes depressed, the body's vital functions also become depressed, and one or another disease can manifest. Consequently, Chinese medicine is essentially a system in which various forms of treatment—everything from acupuncture to diet to herbs—are used to restore the vitality of this underlying essence of existence, the life force itself.

MERIDIANS: CHANNELS OF LIFE ENERGY

The body is traversed by fourteen primary channels of energy, or organ meridians. Ten meridians directly correspond to, and control, the organs of the body, such as the heart and small intestine. (Each meridian will be discussed in depth later in the book.) Twelve of the fourteen primary meridians are bilateral, meaning that a mirror image of each meridian exists on each side of the body. Each of these meridians possesses its own characteristics and precise path and location. Along each meridian is a set of acupressure points that act as tiny charges of energy, which, when pressed or stimulated, set an electromagnetic impulse in motion. That impulse travels along the meridian to the specific organ or function, infusing it with life force and enhancing its function and health. When the life force is strong and balanced, the organ is capable of self-healing. It operates more efficiently, consumes more oxygen, and eliminates accumulated toxins.

When the life force is blocked along these meridians, illnesses arise.

Blocked Qi results in congestion of energy around the blockage and the nearest acupuncture points. This represents an excess of energy near and around the site of the blockage, and deficiencies beyond the blockage. The deficiencies can be quite distant from the blockage itself. Consequently, certain organs will be overstimulated, while others will be deficient, or underactive.

Energy runs along these meridians like a river runs between its banks. If you placed a blockage in the river, let's say a big rock, the area in front of the rock is turbulent and has an overactive flow. Where the river directly encounters the rock, the river is excessive; so, too, is the energy created by the rushing water. Likewise, areas of stagnation appear downstream from the rock; the river is slow-moving and accumulates debris.

It is the same in the human body. When a meridian is blocked, organs downstream, so to speak, of the blockage receive deficient amounts of Qi; those organs will tend to be inactive, stagnant, and will accumulate waste. It's much easier for illness to gain a foothold in these organs. Conversely, the part of the meridian upstream from the blockage will receive excessive amounts of energy, and even backflow, causing certain organs to be overactive and excessive. The job of the acupressurist is to restore balance and harmony by removing the blockage.

Wherever tension and deficiency occurs, sickness will not be far behind. Eventually, it manifests in the lungs, or the reproductive organs, or the breast, or the kidneys, or the lower back, or the stomach, or the liver.

Wherever tension was created in your body and was not resolved or released, it created imbalance and weakness. That is the place you must heal.

In the pages that follow, I'm going to show you how to recognize imbalances and then give you the tools to restore balance.

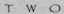

T W O

Yin and Yang

If I were to tell you that one side of a mountain could exist without the other, you'd probably say, "Impossible." Or if I said that at any single moment the entire earth could be bathed in light, without any dark side, you'd disagree. Or if I argued that the animal kingdom could exist indefinitely without male and female, you'd make fast work of my erroneous premise. The fact is that the front side of a mountain could not exist without its back (even if you chopped the mountain in half); a single day is made up of light and dark; and that male and female are needed not only procreate species, but to make things interesting, too.

All of these are examples of the inextricable relationship between yin and yang, the philosophy that forms the foundation of Chinese medicine and, indeed, all of Chinese culture. Simply put, yin and yang are words used to designate all the complementary opposites that make up life—day and night, male and female, winter and summer, autumn and spring, hot and cold, far and near, expansion and contraction, and so forth. The term *yin* is used to describe a general condition characterized by being passive, cool, wet, introverted, and female; *yang* is the general term used to describe characteristics that are more active, hot, dry, extroverted, and male. All of us, no matter what our gender, possess varying degrees of yin and yang characteristics, depending on our native constitutions and current conditions. When yin and yang are balanced within the context of your life and physical condition, you experience health. When they are imbalanced, sickness arises. Through a variety of diagnostic techniques (explained in greater detail in chapter 26) the Chinese were able to determine whether yin or yang was excessive or deficient, thereby causing illness. Once that was established, yin and yang were used as a guide to restoring balance and health. One's overall condition—whether you are excessively yin or yang—will have a direct impact on how Qi flows in your meridians. An excessively cold condition that is contracted, for example, might restrict the flow of Qi along a specific meridian, while too much heat and expansion might cause an excess of energy to flow along a meridian.

While this philosophy is utterly obvious to someone from the East, many Westerners react to the words yin and yang with understandable chagrin. At first glance, yin and yang seem abstract and even mystical. And because so many of us have that reaction, we cannot help but wonder if the application of these foreign words isn't a bit contrived, like forcing an abstruse philosophy on matters that would be far more understandable if approached in another way. Whenever I teach yin and yang, a student will invariably ask me, "Wouldn't it be easier if you just told us that when you see a particular kind of problem, apply this particular method?" They want a formula, a how-to approach to the body. In fact, no such formula exists. Just as every human being is unique, so too are the conditions that each will present to you. Healing is an art—it is the art of making balance, of manipulating yin and yang to establish health.

Let's say a man comes to me with a problem in his lower back, in the area of the midlumbar vertebrae. After examining his back, I find that these vertebrae are drifting to the left side of the body, thus irritating nerves and causing pain. I could focus all my attention on trying to move these vertebrae back into place, but that would be like shoveling sand against the tide. The reason is twofold: First, the muscles in this area—the latissimus dorsi over the kidneys, and the quadratus lumborum, which run along each side of the spine—are loose and empty of tone and vitality. It's as if these muscles and tendons in the lower back lack a certain substance. They are not going to hold the vertebrae in place for any length of time, as is evidenced by the man's condition. The second reason is that the spine is being pulled by a compensatory imbalance and tension elsewhere, which I must now find. I move my hands upward along the back to discover that the trapezius muscles just below the shoulder blades have tremendous tension, especially on the right side of the body. These muscles are overly tight, rigid, hardly movable. This is the compensatory end of the problem that I wrote about in chapter 1. The upper back is loaded with tension and, in general, pulling to the right. The lower back is weak and pulling slightly to the left. To put it another way, the upper back is full, active, externally tense, and yang, while the lower back is empty, loose, internally tense, and yin.

In order to heal the condition, the acupressurist must balance the energy in these areas. To paraphrase Lao Tzu, the acupressurist must empty what is full and fill up what is empty. In practical terms, this means reducing the tension in the upper back—especially the right side—to make the muscles supple, flexible, and capable of a full range of expansion and contraction. Meanwhile, the acupressurist must build up the life force in the lower back, revitalizing the muscles' vitality and tone. Once this is accomplished, the muscles will naturally maintain the normal structure and integrity of the spine. The problem will then be healed.

The acupressurist is working with yin and yang. Because the healer knows yin and yang, he or she is not content just to find the yin place—in this case, the lower back—but searches for the yang compensation, located in this man's upper back. This is the nature of yin and yang: One is never present without the other.

This is a specific example of how healers change the imbalances of yin and yang in the body to restore harmony and health. But in order to make harmony, we must approach each person with an open mind. The more we try to fit people into formulas and compartments, the more we fail to understand them and, in the end, fail to assist the healing process. Each person presents a riddle. Your job is to assess the imbalance and restore harmony to the condition. The best tool for understanding imbalance and restoring harmony is yin and yang.

SEEING THE TWO AND MAKING THEM ONE

As with other epoch-making revelations, the origin of the yin-yang philosophy is shrouded in legend and religious myth. It is said that a great sage, called the Yellow Emperor, was taken up to heaven and instructed in the ways of health, longevity, and an understanding of all phenomena on earth. The essence of this wisdom was the knowledge of yin and yang. His understanding was written down some two thousand years ago and was called the Yellow Emperor's Classic of Internal Medicine (also known as the *Nei Jing*). The Yellow Emperor's Classic is the oldest known medical text in the world.

You might say that the philosophy of yin and yang revealed itself to the Chinese as the foundation of life. Some three thousand years ago—perhaps longer; no one knows for sure—the Chinese observed that all phenomena occurred through a dynamic interplay of opposites. There is no good without evil, no man without woman, no day without night, no high without low, no poor without rich, no sky without earth, no movement without rest, no sickness without health, no health without sickness. Everything that exists does so because of the presence of its opposite.

To a Westerner, each member of these pairs of opposites appears to be a phenomenon, separate from its respective mate. For those of us raised in the West, sickness appears to be a static condition that has taken over the body entirely. People say, "I'm sick." They don't say, "Inside of me, health and illness are having a family argument, but they'll reach a detente soon and I'll go back to being balanced." The latter sentence, while a bit un-wieldy, is nevertheless closer to the way things really are.

If we examine health and illness closely, we soon realize that one never exists without the other. The body is always making some kind of adjust-ment. But even within serious illness, the seeds of health are present and struggling to regain equilibrium and dominance. If that were not the case, no one would recover from anything, including the common cold. Thus, a person who suffers from a cranky stomach can watch what he eats—and avoid greater suffering down the line. The opposite is also true: within health lie the seeds of sickness. We see this all the time in healthy people who are cavalier about their habits because they are healthy which of course makes them sick. As the French say, "A man who can eat everything digs his own grave with his teeth."

No strength exists without weakness, no weakness without the potential for strength. We saw this in the example of our friend with the lower back problem; he had both an overabundance of strength and an exaggerated weakness. Strength and weakness existed side by side—in the same individ-ual.

Westerners are trained to think in absolutes. We are taught to label sit-uations and people as one thing or the other. Often we say that so-and-so "is a good person," or so-and-so "is a bad person," as if any person could be all one or all the other. We are often surprised when apparently contra-dictory information about a situation or a person suddenly appears. We are happy and celebrate when we get a new job or enter into a new relationship, but when we've worked at that job for a while, or gotten to know the person we formerly had such fantasies about, we learn that both the job and our love is a mixed bag—wonderful in many respects, and difficult in others.

For the Chinese, however, contradiction and paradox are the foundations of reality, and therefore to be expected. Indeed, paradox is what makes all of life—and space and time—possible.

Without the relativity of left and right, up and down, near and far, high and low, long and short, infinite and finite, hot and cold, we would be living in a one-dimensional universe. Without polarity, there is no beginning, no middle, and no end. As opposites, yin and yang attract the other and thereby create movement. It is this attraction that makes summer turn into fall and winter, and winter back into summer. It is the attraction of negatively and positively charged particles that creates electricity. It is the powerful allure of the opposite sex that pulls one person toward another. Wherever opposites are, there is movement and change as well.

The knowledge that paradox exists in everything, and that opposites create change, offers us tremendous potential to do good. This knowledge provides us with great power to affect the course of events. For it is precisely because opposites are present in every situation that we have the potential to turn illness into health, and war into peace. Indeed, the fate of any situation depends on our approach to the riddle of yin and yang.

Yin and yang are consistent throughout Chinese philosophy, culture, and art. No matter what Chinese system you use (Five Elements or Eight Principles, for example), yin and yang lie at the foundation. Yin and yang form the basis of all the martial arts, all Oriental approaches to agriculture, social planning, religion, the mystical sciences (such as geomancy and *feng shui*, the art of placement), and divination (the Chinese text, *I Ching* and the Nine Star Ki). They are the common root of all Chinese civilization.

Obviously, if a particular philosophical understanding instructs you on what to do about such practical matters as healing and agriculture, as well as on such esoteric subjects as religion, mystical science, and divination, you have an eminently powerful and widely applicable tool in your hands. It is precisely because yin and yang are present in all matter, all situations, and all of us that it can be applied to every aspect of life—with the results being tremendous insight and instruction on what to do.

By taking up acupressure, you are in fact learning a new way of thinking. I will be challenging you to think of all phenomena as made up of opposites that combine to form a unified whole. Over and over again, and in many different ways, I will be revealing how all of life—every person, every situation, every example of health and illness—is but a manifestation of opposites that are in a state of *temporary* balance or disharmony. In some ways, yin and yang are as intimate to you, the Westerner, as they are to the Chinese. The big difference is that we haven't developed the understanding as deeply as the Chinese have, and we have just begun to apply yin and yang to healing—perhaps its most basic, practical, and natural application.

In order to begin to apply yin and yang to practical situations and especially to healing, let's examine their respective characteristics.

Yin and Yang: An Overview

	YIN	YANG
Density	Contracting Solid	Expanding Diffusing to liquid, fire, and gas
Physical manifestation	Matter	Energy
Type of energy	Potential	Kinetic
Temperament	Dormant Passive Intellectual Following Sleeping	Active Aggressive Physical Leading Awake
Speed	Slow	Fast
Height	Low	High
Body location	Lower parts, to the feet Deep inner organs	Higher parts, to the head Peripheral organs and extremities
Circulation	Blood	Qi
Organs	Dense, internal: kidneys, liver, lungs, heart, spleen	Hollow, superficial: intestines, gall bladder, stomach, bladder
Relative moisture	Moist to saturated	Dry
Time of day	Night	Day
Temperature	Cold	Hot
Distance	Near	Far
Sexual characteristics	Female	Male
Constitution	Female	Male

Direction of transformation	Energy to matter	Matter to energy
	Active to passive	Passive to active
	Male to female	Female to male
	Hot to cold	Cold to hot
	Coalescing	Scattering
	Gathering energy	Burning energy
	Form	Movement

From this chart, you can understand yin and yang in their immediate states—that is, what they represent in any given moment—as well as their respective directions. By direction, I mean how each one is transforming into the other. That is the nature of yin and yang: they attract each other. Each one causes the other to come under its influence, until one opposite has become the other. Yin attracts yang until yang becomes yin. An example of this is the attraction of day to night; after the noon hour, daytime wanes until nighttime dominates. Once that occurs, yang attracts yin, until yin becomes yang—or nighttime gives way entirely to morning and the new light. Let's have a closer look.

YIN AND YANG REVEAL THE DIRECTION OF CHANGE

In its most elemental state, the transformations of yin and yang can be understood as matter (yin) changing into energy (yang), or form (yin) into movement (yang). This, obviously, is a constant and ongoing process. The burning of firewood is an example of wood (in a yin, or solid, condition) being transformed into separated particles of carbon, gas, and heat—all examples of increasing yang.

The reverse is also occurring all the time: Energy is constantly turning into matter; yang is turning into yin.

An example of this is the formation of the physical universe itself. The popular theory on the origins of the universe is the so-called Big Bang, an incomprehensible explosion of energy that was the initial step in the creation of the universe. After Big Bang (or Big Yang, I like to say), hydrogen particles began to gather in spirals to form stars, a yin process. As the particles drew closer together (increasing yin), they began to collide, causing friction and creating heat (yang). Stars, as caldrons of fusion, formed the heavy elements, nitrogen, oxygen, and carbon, which were spread (yang) into the heavens. There, they cooled (yin) and began to gather (more yin) into spirals to form planets and solar systems (even greater yin). One of those solar systems was our own, and one of those planets was Earth. From a relatively gaseous state (yang), the Earth gathered and coalesced to form solid matter (yin) until it became the marvelous jewel that now supports our lives.

This process is a cosmic example of energy becoming matter, and matter becoming energy. This same process takes place all around us, everyday. Iron and steel, for example, form seemingly impervious structures that nonetheless rust; and as they break down, they release the inherent energy that held the molecules together—molecules that combined to form the iron or steel structure. An ordinary apple that sits out on a countertop will begin to brown and break down. Slowly, it shrinks and shrivels up and eventually releases itself into the cosmos as energy. All structures—including our own bodies—eventually give way to energy and movement.

The process is not only in decay, but in regeneration and in life.

Within the human body, matter is continually turning into energy and energy into matter. We consume solid foods (yin), which are chewed, digested, and combusted in our cells—all increasing stages of yang. The energy gives rise to our behavior, also yang. At the same time, we are also turning tiny particles of nutrition and energy into muscle fibers, tissue, and organs—that is, turning yang into yin.

Below is a short chart revealing the manifestations of yin and yang in the human body and human behavior.

YIN	YANG
Catabolism	Metabolism
Assimilation of nutrition	Burning of carbohydrates
Building tissues	Breaking down tissues
Alkalinity	Acidity
Gathering energy	Expending energy
Antioxidation activity	Oxidation
Venous circulation	Arterial circulation
Excessive thinning and release of fluids—urine, sweat, blood	Stagnant blood, lymph, and spinal fluids
Cool temperatures	Fever
Contracted organs, muscles, and tissues	Loose, expanded organs, muscles, and tissues

Silence and introspection	Self-expression
Responding to danger with retreat and inaction	Responding to danger with aggression and action
Thinking	Acting
Becoming matter	Becoming spirit

All these characteristics are *relative* states of yin and yang. I emphasize *relative* because, in our efforts to place labels on conditions or people, we often make the mistake of wanting concrete symptoms or examples of yin and yang.

Yin and yang can be used to measure the greatest extremes we can imagine—which is what people usually associate them with—but they become much more useful when they are used to discern the subtle differences in things.

EIGHT PRINCIPLES OF CHANGE

When yin and yang are applied to the body, they can be defined in even more specific and practical systems. The first one is called the Eight Principles; the second, which I'll discuss later, is called the Five Elements.

When we examine a person's condition from the standpoint of the Eight Principles, we can discern yin and yang as manifesting in the following dualities:

YIN	YANG
Cold	Hot
Empty	Full
Deep	Surface
Imbalanced toward the yin	Imbalanced toward the yang

The last category shows the culmination of the previous conditions. For example, if a person has a fever (hot) and a full feeling in the chest, and the other symptoms are more short-term and acute (obvious and on the surface, such as an acute cold or a hot rash), the condition is imbalanced toward the yang. If, on the other hand, the person is chilled, empty of energy, and in a chronically wasted or hollow state, this person's condition is imbalanced in the yin direction, and will likely be more long-term and chronic.

These two are simple illustrations of overly yin and yang states. Most people suffer from combinations of yin and yang conditions, which we'll talk about more in later chapters.

To apply the Eight Principles to our example of the man with the back problem, I found that his upper back was hot (yang), his lower back cool (yin). His upper back was full (yang), his lower back empty (yin). The tension in the upper back was very much on the surface, like a suit of armor: hard, immovable, and obvious (yang). The tension in the lower back was deep, to the point that it was hard initially to find any strength at all (yin). This will be experienced by the practitioner as a hollow or empty feeling that surrounds knots of tension buried deep within the tissues. In the most general sense, we want to restore balance to these opposing extremes. The extreme yang part must relax and become more supple (or more yin). The extreme yin must become more active, vital, and full (or more yang).

The first step in reestablishing the balance is to work with what is obvious or—as I like to put it—work with what spills over. In the case of our friend, the tension in his upper back was obvious and spilling over; the weakness in his lower back was so apparent that it was obvious and spilling over. This meant that the organs that exist within these regions were also imbalanced. This is an important point because we are not only working with the surface tension in Integrative Acupressure, but with the corresponding organs and meridians that supply these organs with Qi.

This is made possible, in part, because the regions of our body develop together prenatally. As we develop in our mothers' wombs, individual organs, the nerves that supply these organs, the muscles that support them, and the acupuncture meridians that provide life force to them all develop in unison. Thus, the kidneys, the nerves that supply the kidneys, the muscles that support them, and the kidney and bladder meridians all develop simultaneously, as one unified aspect of the body. All the other parts of the body do the same, and thus an intimate relationship is established that remains intact for life. Problems with one member of this four-part harmony (organs, nerves, muscles, and meridians) are symptomatic of problems with the other three. Conversely, to work with one member is to work with all four. Yet we never forget the whole, which means that one problem will affect the rest of the body in the form of compensatory imbalances. You might say that the whole is the fifth aspect of this circular healing process.

When we apply this understanding to our example, we recognize that problems with the man's lower and upper back corresponded to problems in specific organs. That meant that his kidneys (corresponding to the lower back) and the liver (corresponding to the mid back) were troubled. Thus, when I began to work on the lower back, I would be working to establish the strength in the kidneys, making them more yang. When I worked on his mid back, I'd be working with his liver, dispersing the excess and making it more yin.

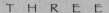

Working on the Body

*Once a beginning acupressur-*ist starts to understand yin and yang, he or she immediately wants to correct all the imbalances in a person's body overnight. The novice thinks the whole process is simple: "All I have to do," he says, "is get down beneath the tension, stimulate the acupuncture points, and start galvanizing the body with Qi." Reality, unfortunately, is a little more complicated.

The body is a series of layers. Each layer must be treated with gentleness and great respect. You must gain the trust of the person you are working on. But more importantly, you must gain the trust of his or her body, which is reacting to your touch, your technique, and the respect that flows through your hands. A client may say that he or she trusts you long before he or she actually does. But the body doesn't lie; it's not polite; and it won't let you get to its secrets and heal its imbalances if it doesn't trust your methods, your intention, and your abilities.

Therefore, I always tell my students: Treat a client's body as if you are asking the body for its permission to do your job. The client may have come to you because he heard you were good, and he may pay you well, but that means little or nothing to the client's body, which on one hand wants desperately to protect its imbalances and adaptations. On the other hand, the body wants to surrender those imbalances and be free and healthy once again. You must show the body the way to do that.

When you begin your work, therefore, you must move carefully into the depths of the body, into each of its layers. Long before you actually reach the acupuncture point and start to stimulate the flow of Qi along the meridian and to the organ itself, you will have confronted two other layers of tissue and energy.

As you begin to explore your client's body, you will find places that might be characterized as "full" or that give a sense of "fullness." These full places may seem at first to be hard, or swollen, or taut with tension. There may be little or no clarity or definition in these large masses of tension. As you search, say, the lower back, you will find other places that seem "empty." Upon closer examination, you'll discover that within an "empty" place lies an island—or islands—of contracted tissue. The empty space surrounding this island of tension feels loose and even a little watery. The island itself feels like it's balled up and tight.

The question will arise in your mind: Where should I begin working, on the large masses of tension, or the little balls of tension inside the empty spaces? The answer is to start with the large masses of tension, the places where there is a lack of clarity. Disperse the tension, while gently sending some of that tension toward the "empty" spaces you also discovered. In this way, the blood, lymph, and Qi will flow in the direction of the empty places, the places where the body is weak. Blood carries oxygen, immune cells, and nutrition to tissues. Lymph, a fluid that contains immune cells, proteins, and fats, travels throughout the body via a vast network of lymph vessels and nodes. Lymph removes waste from tissues and brings it to the bloodstream, where the waste products can be neutralized by the liver and eliminated from the body. (See chapter 21 for more on the lymph system.) Qi, of course, is the fundamental life force, which enables the body to function. In the weak or empty places these fluids and Qi will start the healing process.

RELEASING THE POINT AND MERIDIAN FROM TENSION

The first layer of tissue is a flat surface of tension. There is little or no definition to this surface. It feels like a hard, impenetrable wall. There are no lumps or bumps. This area may feel like one big sheet of tension with skin stretched over it. The skin and subcutaneous tissue may feel loose or that they're adhering to it. It can even feel like loose sand on top of sedimentary rock. That rock is the layer of surface tension I am talking about.

This is the layer that is most typically worked on by therapeutic massage practitioners, such as in Swedish or Esalen massage. Your instinct may be to fight this rocklike wall or try to knock it down. Don't. The body will recoil and establish an even greater armor against your work. Gently move into the tension and release it by massaging and moving it. Imagine that you are working with cold clay that, with the work of your hands, begins to get warm and more pliable. With time and consistent work, it will begin to give way, gradually revealing another layer below. This process is what I call "releasing," and this is a term that I will use consistently from chapter 4 onward.

That which lies below the layers of tension are bands of muscle—often in spasm—that can be felt radiating up and down or across. These muscle fibers can feel like strings, wires, or even fat cords, depending on the type of muscle involved and the amount of tension. However, as a general guide, the thicker ropes tend to be at the surface, while the thinner strings or wires are found at the deeper levels. These thinner strings are revealed to your hands as you release the upper layers of tension. Many deep-tissue body-workers deal at the level of bands and cords. Among the most common of such practices are Rolfing and Neuromuscular Therapy.

As you work deeper and release the tension from these cords, you begin to feel individual knots. These are the acupuncture points. Often, they feel like large knots, or bunches of energy and tension. These gradually become smaller and smaller with continued work until they become tiny points of energy. You must unravel the knots by—again—being gentle, sure, and healing. This is the third and deepest layer, the level of the meridians and acupuncture points, and the level most commonly worked on by acupuncture, acupressure, and myotherapy.

With experience you will find that, as you progress through the layers, your fingers are invariably drawn to these points. They cannot stay away. There is a mystery here, a dynamic energy that is encapsulated in whatever armoring the person has thrown up. The point exists like pure energy, like light below the darkness of tension and conflict. But it cannot be forced out. It must be gently coaxed. The energy must be allowed to meet you halfway, because the person must release the tension that stands guard over the acupuncture point. Your purpose is to help the person learn how to release that tension. Rather than forcing the release, together you are teaching the body to release the tension on its own. Consequently, you want to work gently on the tension until the body permits you to go to the next layer.

MOVING THE ENERGY WITH YOUR TOUCH

Your thumbs and fingers can move in a circular pattern or in short strokes across the area. From time to time, you should disperse the tension surrounding the area by enlarging the circle and then stroking the tissue away from the area, as though clearing whatever tension you've dislodged.

As the area opens and releases, it becomes more defined, more characteristic, more precise in its nature. The point is revealed and it is full of energy. It feels almost like water flowing through your hands. The moment the area releases, there is a kind of satisfaction that is transmitted to you. This part of the body is alive again in a way that it wasn't just twenty minutes ago.

It may take several sessions to get certain areas to release substantially. The areas slowest to release, of course, suffer the greatest problems and are at the core of the person's long-term imbalance. To the practitioner, this progression is like going back through time, excavating deeper and deeper layers of trauma.

Use this same gentle but persistent technique as you move through the layers of the tension, to the muscle below, and then finally to the points themselves.

To apply these same ideas to our example in chapter 2—the man who came to me with a back problem—I begin by working on the upper back gently but firmly, loosening the tension on the surface. At first, I do this by finding a particularly full, impenetrable area—a place where muscle tension has accumulated in a tight fist or spiral—and dispersing the energy outward and downward toward the empty area. I run my fingers from the place where an acupuncture point is located, a point over which there is considerable tension, and then move the tension away from that point. Initially, all I can do is to work at this surface layer of tension. His body hasn't learned to trust me enough yet to allow me to go below the armoring that he has established. Nevertheless, I know that other problems exist below the tension. Getting down to those lower layers will take some time—often two to three hour-long sessions. Meanwhile, I am content to disperse the upper layers of energy. Eventually, I will have to get down to those lower levels to address the deeper imbalance. The image is one of digging in sand; if I dig too deeply, the walls cave in. If all I do is clear the surface, I will never make a deep change.

As I release the tension, I envision myself moving some of that excess strength of the upper back into the area of weakness, his lower back. What I am really doing, however, is allowing the circulation of nerve impulses, blood, and Qi that were stuck in the upper back—and especially in the area of the liver—to move freely into the kidney area once again. This will help to build up the area that is weak—even before I begin to work on it directly with my hands.

When I have dissolved some of the tension in the upper back, I move down to the lumbar region and the area of the kidneys. When I had first put my hands on this man's lower back and discovered the obvious emptiness in this area, I realized that the muscles, nerves, and kidneys were all deficient, or lacking in Qi. The obvious symptom of such a state is that the area is empty, or yin, with distinct knots and bands. The whole area cannot hold adequate life force to support the organs, the nerves, and the muscles. Hence, the area is weak, which is one of the reasons the integrity of the spine has broken down. It is my job to build up the Qi, blood circulation, and lymph in a part of the body that has degenerated. Correcting the spine will be almost a by-product of the larger job I am seeking to accomplish.

Gently, I probe the weakened kidney area. In general it is flaccid, but as I probe deeper and finally go to the kidney points themselves, I find them tight, hard, and cold. They are like two knots surrounded by emptiness. All the energy of the lower back has collected inside the kidneys. The life force has retreated into these two organs. This is one reason why the area is deficient.

Thus, it is immediately clear what I have to do with this man's back. First, I must release the surface tension on the upper back so that the muscles stop pulling on the upper spine. The release of the surface tension will also allow blood and lymph to flow more freely to the tissues and organs below. Once he allows me to go below his armoring, I begin to stimulate specific acupuncture points with my fingers which pump life force into his liver, an organ that in this man's case is congested, excessively yang, and stagnant. This process gradually heals the upper part of the back.

At the same time, I work with his lower back. Gradually and gently, I begin to move the trapped energy out of the kidneys and back into the nerves and muscles of the region. Once I get the kidneys to relax and release—to let go of the Qi they are holding—I also stimulate specific acupuncture points and meridians, especially the bladder and kidney meridians, to bring Qi to the kidneys, bladder, and the rest of the body. As the kidneys release energy and as I draw more Qi to the region—including to the organs themselves—the lower back begins to regain its strength. It begins to feel fuller and more responsive to my touch. Gradually, it shows clear signs of healing. Generally, the person feels a distinct improvement after the first or second treatment, but it may take anywhere from six to ten sessions to truly reestablish balance and health in a badly injured back. (More on the back in chapters 19 and 20.)

As the body heals, its natural integrity begins to reestablish itself. Our posture and the positioning of every vertebra—indeed, every bone and muscle—exists in a kind of blueprint in the brain. By removing the excess tension and restoring health to the organs that lie below the tension, the body relaxes and its natural posture asserts itself. In the case of our friend with the back problem, gradually the muscles once again support the spine equally from the left and the right sides of the body. The spine straightens itself and all of his symptoms disappear.

Without tools or understanding, we cannot penetrate the surface to see below, into the depths of a situation. By understanding yin and yang, you will have the key to understanding what lies below the surface.

You understand that no strength exists without weakness, no weakness without a corresponding strength. Very often, a person's true health condition is disguised by an apparent weakness or strength that's covering over an opposite condition that lies below, or elsewhere in the body. To know yin and yang and to have the ability to apply it to the human body is to have the keys to health itself.

LOW-BACK PAIN

A seventy-year-old man came to see me suffering from long-standing, chronic low-back pain. Healthy and vital overall, his problem originated because he spent a lot of time sitting in chairs and driving his car, which put excessive pressure on his lower back. He also suffered from chronic tension, which had accumulated in his upper back and shoulders. What finally brought him to me was that he had recently injured his lower back and, after months of seeing chiropractors, an orthopedist, a physical therapist, and a Neuromuscular Therapist—all with no improvement—he decided to try acupressure.

The problem was in the lower lumbar area, where he had significant inflammation around the lumbar 4 and lumbar 5 vertebrae. This was being exacerbated by too little curvature in the upper lumbar area, caused by stagnant Qi in the kidney points, which was itself brought about by long-term stress. With the upper lumbar curving too little, the lower lumbar compensated by curving too much. The first thing I did was release the tension and stagnant Qi in the upper lumbar area, using the dispersal method. Gradually, I got the upper lumbar area to relax and let go of the stagnant Qi. I then distributed that Qi to the lower lumbar area, where I worked to improve the curve of the lower lumbar spine. I also cleared the whole bladder meridian on the back and behind the legs, to allow the free flow of Qi. Especially important was the point behind the knee called Bladder 40, which released the entire back. This boosted Qi throughout the back, thus strengthening the entire spinal column and the muscles, meridians, and points along the spine.

After two weeks (four treatments), the man was out of pain and so much better that he told me he was ready to go to a very important trade show. I advised against the trip, but he insisted that it was essential. Sure enough, the following Monday, after the show, he called me to say that he was in terrible pain. He had reinjured his lower back.

Once again I worked extensively on his back, relaxing and releasing the upper back and distributing Qi in the lower back, where it was weak. Within a few weeks, he was well again. This time he followed my advice and proceeded cautiously. We worked on his back for a few months, after which he was entirely out of pain, his muscles were stronger, his upper lumbar had released, and the curve in his lower lumbar area was restored to normal. He could now conduct business without restriction.

FOUR

Meridians

In the fourteen chapters that follow this one, I will be showing you how you can use acupressure to heal yourself or someone else. But before we can apply the practice, we must first go over some key techniques and terms that will be used throughout the next section of the book.

MERIDIANS: THE ROOTS OF ORGANS

The yin organs—liver, lung, spleen, kidney, heart, and pericardium (the sac that surrounds and protects the heart)—are deep in the body and share a common purpose: altering, circulating, and storing blood and Qi. The yang organs—gall bladder, large intestine, stomach, small intestine, bladder, and Triple Warmer (the three zones of energy in the torso)—are closer to the surface and are part of the digestive system.

As you might expect, no organ operates independently in the meridian network. In fact, each yin organ and its meridian works in tandem with a corresponding yang organ and meridian. In chapter 25, we will explore more fully how these pairs function together as part of the Five Elements. Let's begin our work now at using acupressure to heal.

Keep in mind that when you work on a specific meridian, you are working on a related organ as well. Meridians are the energetic roots of organs. As with the roots of a plant, the meridians draw nourishment—in this case, Qi—into the pathway and then send it on to the organ. The meridians draw the Qi from the outer environment. Qi originates from many sources, among the most important of which are cosmic and solar rays that radiate down upon the earth and upon each of us. In addition, there is also the earth's own electromagnetic body that surrounds and permeates our planet and bathes all of us in its energy. All living things—indeed, every object on earth—are continuously being bathed in Qi from all of these sources. There is no limit to the life force that flows to us. The only limits are those created by the ways we think, the emotions we experience, the foods and liquids we ingest, and the ways in which we behave.

Qi is also boosted along the meridian and to the organ whenever we press or stimulate an acupressure point, which in turn sends a charge of electromagnetic energy along the meridian to the organ. Every cell and organ in the body is dependent upon life force flowing to it along the meridian. In the same way, all healing depends upon an abundant flow of life force, or Qi, to every cell and organ of the body. By raising the amount of Qi flowing to an organ, you can boost its vitality, dynamism, and capacity to self-heal.

Acupressure points serve as batteries, or tiny sources of Qi, within the body.

TREATING THE POINTS, MERIDIANS, AND ORGANS

The methods you will use to heal yourself or someone else are point and meridian release, Shu points, alarm points, foot reflexology, and direct organ release. I'll give a brief introduction to each of the forms; then, in successive chapters, we will learn to use them one at a time with each meridian and organ pair. Use the technique for releasing the point and for probing the layers of tissue that I described in chapter 3. I'll summarize point and meridian release briefly below.

Points are found at very precise locations along the line of energy, or pathway, that is the meridian. Points are actually very specific sites that, when stimulated, generate Qi flow along the meridian. Dr. Becker, the researcher I mentioned in chapter 1, found that these points generate direct current along the meridian pathway. By increasing energy along the meridian, healing is promoted.

The most powerful points for long-term change are considered to be those on the extremities, meaning the points at the hands, feet, below the knees, and below the elbows. Whenever you release an organ, you should first massage these points and then move toward the body. Whenever you encounter an acupressure point, you will likely find it in a depression between tendons, muscles, or in the bone. As you stimulate it, you will likely discover one or another of the following conditions: empty or full, tight or loose, hot or cool, sensitive or painful.

As you become more familiar with the points, you will recognize immediately a kind of electrical feedback that will emanate from the point as soon as you put your fingers on it. If you are new to acupressure, you may not recognize this electrical feedback immediately. Do not be concerned. With time, you will become increasingly sensitive and knowledgeable about the location of points. With just a little experience, you'll have a palpable sensation of electrical energy the instant you put your hand or fingertips on another person, even when the person is wearing heavy clothing.

Incidentally, the full name of each point is often abbreviated using a letter or two from the name of the organ (e.g., LV for liver, SI for small intestine) followed by the number of the point.

RELEASING A POINT OR MERIDIAN

Releasing an acupressure point simply means to remove a blockage or tension that exists within the point or along the meridian. Very often a point is buried below layers of tension when you first place your hand on it, or the point may be closed. If either of these conditions exists, gently work through the layers, using the circular movements as discussed in chapter 3. If the point is closed, it may feel dull or emit a very weak charge. Your goal is to get it to open, to stimulate Qi from the point, and to make it more sensitive and receptive to the Qi that is flowing to the point from the environment.

You can assist the relaxation of the point by slowly sliding your thumb across the point while pivoting your thumb so that you are still on the point.

ACUTE AND CHRONIC BLOCKAGES

The blockage may be in an acute or a chronic phase. An *acute* phase arises when the body is addressing the blockage or injury and is attempting to heal the disorder. In general, acute conditions are usually sensitive and even painful; they are sometimes inflamed and frequently hot. When the blockage is *chronic*, the condition is generally older and the body has accommodated itself to the injury. Generally, a compensatory pattern—such as an imbalanced way of walking (a limp, for example) or bending or reaching for an object— has developed to keep the body from feeling the pain or injury. Acupressure points that are in a chronic phase are often buried under tissue—a condition I refer to as armoring; they are often cool and difficult to find.

To release a point, apply moderate pressure with your finger or fingers—usually one or both thumbs are used. Remember, the purpose of the release is to stimulate Qi along the meridian and allow the point to relax, so it is important to begin gently and then work at a deeper level as the person's body begins to open up and trust you.

MEASURING DISTANCES TO FIND POINTS

Our unit of measure is called a "finger-width," (or simply "finger"). One finger-width is about the width of the last segment of your index finger.

For example, let's find Large Intestine 4 and 5. LI 4 is found within the great muscle between the thumb and index finger, close to the joint that is formed by the thumb and index finger bones. LI 5 is in the depression in the wrist, at the very root of the thumb. It is approximately three "finger-widths" up from LI 4.

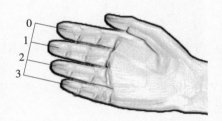

MEASURING FINGER DISTANCES

SHU POINTS

The Shu points are found at about two inches to the left and right of the spine, along the bladder meridian.

KEY TO THE SHU POINTS CHART

Listed on the following pages are the labels for each point on the Shu points chart, along with their corresponding Bladder meridian points and associated symptoms. The inner points on the chart are the actual Shu points, while the outer points hold additional Qi which may overflow from

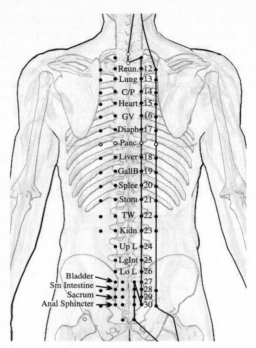

The Shu Points on the Bladder Meridian

the Shu points. These points can become tight or irritated when long-term congestion occurs in the Shu points.

Reun—Bl 12: The Reunion point serves as a nexus for all the Yang meridians. If it is tight, it shows deficiency.

Lung—Bl 13: Becomes congested or "knotted" when the lungs are deficient or irritated.

C/P—Bl 14: Circulation/Pericardium point. Becomes congested when the nervous system and heart become stressed.

Heart—Bl 15: Becomes blocked when the nervous system and heart are stressed.

GV—Bl 16: Governing Vessel. Becomes tense when the central nervous system and spinal cord are chronically stressed.

Diaph—Bl 17: Diaphragm point. Becomes congested when the diaphragm is tight or the nervous system becomes irritated, or with deficient blood conditions (see chapter 26 on Chinese Diagnosis).

Panc—Pancreas point: This is not considered a standard point in Chinese acupuncture, but I have found that this point is a good diagnostic tool to determine the condition of the pancreas. Specifically, this point becomes tight whenever the pancreas is inflamed.

Liver—Bl 18: Becomes tight or swollen when the liver is congested or irritated.

Gall B—Bl 19: Gall Bladder. Becomes tight or swollen when the gall bladder is congested or irritated.

Splee—Bl 20: Spleen. Becomes tight or swollen when the spleen and digestive system are deficient or irritated.

Stom—Bl 21: Stomach. Becomes tight or swollen when the stomach is irritated.

TW—Bl 22: Triple Warmer. In Integrative Acupressure, we relate this point to the adrenal glands. Tension here indicates physical or emotional stress.

Kidn—Bl 23: Kidney. Becomes tight or swollen when the kidneys are deficient or irritated.

Up L—Bl 24: Upper Lumbar point. Becomes tight or swollen when there is congestion or irritation in the small of the back.

LgInt—Bl 25: Large Intestine. Becomes tight or swollen when the large intestines are congested or irritated.

Lo L—Bl 26: Lower Lumbar point. Becomes tight or swollen when there is congestion or irritation of the small of the back.

Bladder—Bl 27: Bladder point. Becomes tight or swollen when there is deficiency or irritation of the bladder.

Sm Intestine—Bl 28: Small Intestine. Becomes tight or swollen when there is congestion or irritation of the small intestines.

Sacrum—Bl 29: Sacrum and sacroiliac joint. Becomes tight or swollen when there is congestion or irritation of the sacral area.

Anal Sphincter—Bl 30: Anal sphincter point. Becomes tight or swollen when there is congestion or irritation of the anal sphincter, which tightens the anus to prevent defecation.

Shu points direct Qi or life force directly into the organ to which they are related, and for this reason they are important points in any treatment.

The Small Intestine Shu point, for example, will send a powerful charge of life force into the small intestine whenever the point is stimulated.

There are two ways you can work with the Shu points. One is to release the entire back, using the Shu points as an aid in diagnosis and treatment; the other is to go to the particular Shu point for an organ you are working with (which is what we will do in the following chapters).

Shu points are often sensitive, tight, or swollen (or full) or empty when the organ has been deprived of Qi for some time and now suffers from some degree of imbalance. If the point is in an acute phase, it may be swollen (or inflamed, and thus very acute), soft, and quite sensitive, even painful.

As the imbalance becomes more chronic, the point will become more tight, more resistant to your efforts at releasing it. In time, the point will become harder to find, and increasingly armored with tense muscle or indistinct tissue. At this stage, the point will feel as if it is very dense and spread out over a large area. (Once you have worked with the area for a while, you'll find that tension begins to emerge as lines and points.) Many men have very dense, thick backs, as if they have a layer of thick, indistinct muscle and fat covering their backs. This indicates long-term chronic conditions and Shu points that are insensitive and unable to promote optimal Qi flow to organs.

WHEN WORKING ON YOURSELF

Obviously, it will be difficult for you to reach and open some of your own Shu points, simply because you will not be able to reach. In that case, put a couple of tennis balls in a sock, place the sock on the floor, and roll on top of the balls along your spine. Do this slowly and gently, and it will eventually open your Shu points.

ALARM POINTS

Alarm points, also called Mu points in Chinese medicine, are simply that: They let you know the organ and the particular point it is associated with is imbalanced because they are inordinately sensitive when touched, or emit an inordinate amount of pain when probed, even superficially.

A good alarm point example is the stomach alarm, halfway between the navel and the sternum. It will become painful with the classic stomachache. Alarm points usually show a relative excess of energy, and are associated with acute conditions. Of course, if an organ remains acutely irritated long enough, the point will eventually become chronically tight and sensitive to deeper pressure, indicating a more chronic condition.

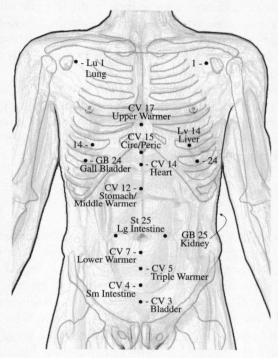

THE ALARM POINTS

SOURCE POINTS

In the chapters that follow, I will frequently refer to source points, which, when stimulated, balance the Qi that flows within the related meridian. If excess energy is within the meridian, stimulation of the source point will disperse and calm the energy flowing within that pathway. If the meridian is deficient of Qi, stimulation of the source point will promote the flow of additional Qi along the meridian. The source point, therefore, is a kind of regulating point, harmonizing imbalances and thereby relieving symptoms.

REFLEXOLOGY

Reflexology, which is fully discussed in chapter 24, is the use of acupressure on specific points located on the feet that correspond to organs throughout the body. Virtually all the work is done on the bottoms of the feet. The left side of each foot corresponds to the left side of the body, and the right side of each foot with the right side of the body. Thus, they are not mirror images of each other. The toes are used to stimulate the head region and nervous system; the arch of the foot corresponds with the spine; and the heels with the pelvis.

By working on the areas associated with a particular organ or structure, you will be able to find any tight or painful spots that would indicate an imbalance. Massaging the area will affect the organ or structure it represents. Although we usually need to use deep pressure with reflexology, it should not be a really painful process.

ORGAN RELEASE

One of the best ways we can assess an organ and optimize its functioning is to massage the organ itself. In general, we can apply the same concepts of fullness and emptiness, chronic and acute, to the organs. For example, by probing the right side of the body, just below the rib cage, you can determine the condition of the liver. If the liver is swollen, or full, as it is for many people today, even the most gentle probing will be felt as discomfort or mild pain by your client. If probing actually feels good to the client—deeper probing feels better for many people—the liver is empty and deficient. Obviously, when probing the digestive tract, you must take into account when the person last ate and whether or not the stomach or intestines are full. Yet another reason to begin gently.

Whenever you encounter acute inflammation in an organ or area, you can be pretty sure that something is irritating the organ, such as an allergen, toxin, pathogenic organism, injury, or muscle tension caused by stress. Massage the organ very gently and dispersively to move the excess Qi and tension away from the organ. If the acute inflammation is sustained long enough, it will eventually become chronic. Here, we will need to work deeper to release the congestion.

For the most part, organ massage is not a necessity, because you can stimulate the key points and meridians, especially at the extremities. This is especially important when the organ is very tender, imbalanced, or suffering from some type of disorder. By releasing the meridian from the extremities, you can begin and nurture the healing process.

Obviously, it doesn't seem practical to massage certain organs, namely the heart and lungs. Even with these organs, however, we can release or disperse through mobilizing the rib cage.

BEFORE YOU BEGIN WORKING, CENTER YOURSELF

One of the challenges every bodyworker faces is maintaining a balanced and professional relationship with his or her clients, which means the practitioner must avoid taking on the various kinds of tension and imbalances that clients arrive with. A bodyworker forms a personal relationship with each client, and it's easy to be affected quite viscerally by the relationship. Centered breathing is a tool for keeping balance.

In the early years of my practice, a friend who lived several hours away organized a weekend in which I was to give acupressure treatments for twelve hours a day. I had never before attempted to treat so many people at once. By the middle of Saturday afternoon, I was exhausted and I felt I couldn't possibly continue. Still, I felt obligated to go on. I prayed for help and suddenly remembered a Daoist meditative exercise. I began by drawing energy in through the top of my head, and down my back into the abdomen, then exhaled upward through my abdomen and chest. I repeated this breathing exercise for the next twenty minutes or more, concentrating on filling myself with Qi. Within a half hour, I felt miraculously rejuvenated.

The rest of the weekend flew by, and I did some of the best acupressure I had ever done. I continued to feel energetic for several days. Over the years this exercise, called centered breathing, has helped me in a variety of situations.

I especially recommend that you do this exercise at the beginning of every day, and whenever your work becomes extremely demanding and you find your energy and concentration waning.

CENTERED BREATHING

Get into a comfortable sitting position and touch GV 20, which is located at the back of the top of the head on the midline. Now rest your hand at your side again, and close your eyes. Breathe in through your nose and out through your mouth, while touching the tip of your tongue to the front of the roof of your mouth, just behind your teeth. This connects the Conception and Governing Vessels. As you breathe out, you can let your tongue rest.

Stay aware of that point, GV 20, and imagine that, as you breathe in, you are drawing energy in through the point, over the back of your head and down your back until it reaches the kidney area. As you reach your full breath, imagine the energy swirling around in your abdomen, in the bowl of your pelvis. Then, as you breathe out, move the energy up through your abdomen, chest, neck, and out your mouth. Repeat the above cycle, imagining the energy moving as a stream through your body.

Now try to follow the energy carefully as it moves through your body. Do you feel areas that are blocked or tight? Allow the breath to keep moving through your body and spend some time getting to know one of these areas. Don't try to unblock it, just try to become more familiar with the area. Get a clear picture of where it is in your body—how far up and down, how far to each side, how deep into your body. If you held it in your hands, what would it feel like? Would it be cold or warm? Hard or soft? Would its surface be rough or smooth? What color would it be? Again, try to get a clear picture of where it is in your body. What you'll notice is that the clearer you picture the area, the more it changes—it gets smaller and softer.

Get back in touch with your breathing. You haven't stopped the meditation; you have allowed your unconscious to continue it. Become aware of it. Now imagine that, as the breath moves through the area of congestion, it is like little fingers sweeping the tension away. As you reach your full breath, feel it swirl around like mist or smoke, then breathe it out through the abdomen, chest, throat, and mouth. Feel the breath swirling around the area of blockage, dislodging any tension, relaxing the muscles, and bringing oxygen to the tissues. Breathe out the tension, let it go.

When you are working with a client, you can use this same breathing technique with a minor variation. Instead of having the energy go out through your mouth, direct it through your arms and into the person. In the same way that you felt blockages in yourself, you can feel blockages in your client wherever you don't feel the energy moving freely. Practice this every time you work on yourself or another person. It can make a dramatic difference in your ability to release an area and in your own comfort.

This exercise activates the "Great Central Channel"—the conception and governing vessels—which runs along the midline of the body and balances all the meridians. In addition, breathing in "Heaven's Qi" through the Great Central Channel increases the energy flow throughout your body, and the body of your client.

Inevitably, you will forget the meditation while you're working. Rather than thinking that you have to start up again, get in touch with your breathing. As long as you are breathing, you are still circulating energy. If you create an image in your subconscious mind of drawing energy inward with every breath, centered breathing will become a part of your life and you will seldom have to think about it.

Liver Meridian

We live in a world filled with poisons, many of which have the power to destroy us. One of our greatest defenders is the largest of our internal organs, the liver, which identifies and neutralizes virtually every toxin we encounter. Each and every day, your liver literally saves your life. It also serves us in more subtle, yet essential ways. Unlike the Western approach to the human body, which sees the organs from purely a biological and physiological viewpoint, the Chinese see the human body in both the physical and the metaphorical sense. The liver is regarded as the "commanding general" of the body because, along with the liver meridian, it regulates Qi flow throughout the body. When looked at in this larger context, the liver takes on much more dramatic dimensions. While the kidneys are considered the root of the will, and the heart the reservoir of our innate nature, the liver provides us with the capacity to express both—the will and the inherent talents and abilities that reside within us.

A healthy liver, therefore, is essential to both our survival and our enjoyment of life. Acupressure provides the tool for you to strengthen and restore the health of your liver.

Common Physical Symptoms of Imbalance
Red face (excess Qi)

Pale, drawn face (deficient Qi)

Menstrual pain, irregularity, blood clotting, PMS

Pain and swelling in genitals

Headaches at the top of the head

Migraines

Dizziness

Disorders of the eye and vision

Muscle spasms, seizures, convulsions

Pale fingernails, ridges in nails, cracked nails

Tendon-related pain or disorders

Allergies

Easily bruised

Dandruff and hair loss

Common Emotional Symptoms of Imbalance

Anger (excess Qi)

Frustration (excess Qi)

Depression (deficient Qi)

Lack of will (deficient Qi)

There are several steps to strengthening the organ. These include clearing the meridian and stimulating specific points. After you've cleared the meridian, you can use the alarm point to disperse excess energy and the Shu point to boost energy within the organ. You can assess both the alarm and Shu points to determine the extent to which the organ is imbalanced.

THE LIVER: FROM WEST AND EAST

The liver is the largest of all internal organs, spanning from the right side of the body, directly beneath the rib cage, to the left side, directly below the left nipple. It is cone-shaped—wider on the right side and narrowing the farther you track it to the left.

The liver is a living laboratory, producing an array of complex and essential chemicals. Among them are: bile acids, used to break up and digest fats; proteins, such as albumin, which regulate water exchange between cells; coagulant, which makes blood clot; and globulin, which combines with iron to carry oxygen in the blood. The liver also produces immune constituents, such as complement, which fights infection, and more than a thousand enzymes used for digestion and assimilation of nutrition.

As if this were not enough, the liver produces cholesterol—both the "good" cholesterol, called HDL, and the "bad," or LDL—and takes fat and cholesterol out of the blood.

In addition, the liver identifies the chemicals each of us ingests via air, water, and food, and it neutralizes any substance that it regards as poisonous to the human body. For this reason, the liver is regarded in both Western and Eastern medicine as a blood-purifying organ. At any one time, the liver holds as much as 25 percent of the body's blood supply within the organ.

In Chinese medicine, the liver and the liver meridian are considered the controller of the life force. The liver and its meridian are most closely associated with expression of the will, or willpower, and with creativity. When life energy is weak, it very often means the liver is troubled or weakened itself.

The liver provides blood and Qi flow to tendons, muscles, ligaments, nails, and the eyes. This blood and Qi flow allow for the ability to enjoy deep sleep, emotional balance, especially regarding anger, and balanced Qi flow to all the meridians.

FINDING AND TREATING THE LIVER MERIDIAN

To restore harmony and health to the liver and the liver meridian (Lv), Qi flow must be reestablished to the organ and within the electromagnetic pathway. To do that, we must stimulate key points along the meridian.

The liver meridian begins at a point by the inside of the big toenail, passes over the top of the foot, continues above the inside of the ankle, runs past the inside of the knee and along the inner thigh. It proceeds through the genital region, upward to the sides of the body, and then to the ribs, just over the liver (for the meridian on the right side of the body) and just over the spleen (on the left side).

When working on the liver meridian, we are addressing both acute (short-term) obstructions to the flow of Qi and chronic (long-term) blockages that reflect a deep, internal imbalance. Points in an acute condition are more tender and sensitive and will announce themselves—either as pain or heat or as inflammation—almost immediately upon your touch. Points that have been blocked chronically can be more difficult to find, but in any case exist below layers of tension and congestion. (See chapter 4 for a fuller explanation of acute and chronic conditions.)

Remember, as you work gently with either acute or chronic points, you are using yin and yang to disperse areas that are excessive and to build up areas that are deficient.

You can release your own liver meridian. Many Shu points can only be reached with a partner, or by placing two tennis balls in a sock, placing them on the floor, and then gently rolling your back over the balls.

The most important points on the liver meridian are found between the knees and elbows. By treating the points described next, you will clear the meridian.

RELEASING THE LIVER MERIDIAN

Begin by tracing the meridian with your hand. Once you know your way, you can come back and massage any sensitive points. Then, as described in chapters 3 and 4, you will "release" the meridian by applying moderate pressure on the sensitive point, using the release and dispersal technique, until the tension dissipates and the energy flows from the point once again.

Begin by massaging the meridian on the outer side of the big toe, at the base of the nail. Move your hands methodically and firmly toward the ankle along the meridian line at the top of the foot. Move your hand toward the ankle to Liver 3, located at the very apex of the V formed by the two tendons of the big toe and the index toe. Massage firmly, but gently. This is the "source" point on the liver meridian, which can balance the liver Qi and restore energy along the meridian. Check for congestion or sensitivity here; massage the point gently, and return to it later if it needs further work. Liver 3 also can be used to release blockages found elsewhere along the meridian.

From here, move up the foot to the ankle, between the two tendons just to the inside of the very front of the ankle. This is Liver 4.

Find the center of the medial malleolus (the peak of the ankle); put your little finger on it, while placing your other fingers along the inside of the shinbone (the tibia) so that your index finger is the closest to the knee. Allow each finger to lightly touch the finger next to it. (Although there are four fingers touching, this is still referred to as a three-finger distance; the first finger is not counted.)

About two-fifths up the inside of the leg from the medial malleolus, along the tibia, is Spleen 6. Often, there is a little notch in the sharp edge of the bone where the point can be found. It is a very sensitive and very important point because three meridians—the liver, spleen, and kidney meridians—can be balanced by stimulating the point. Spleen 6 is usually quite sensitive; massage it with care.

From here, massage forward one finger just onto the flat of the bone, and massage up toward the knee three fingers to find Lv 5 and, at six fingers, Lv 6. Next move behind the bone into the calf muscle, massaging up toward the knee about two fingers behind the bone. (You can massage with your index finger while keeping your middle finger between the index and the edge of the bone.) Where your index finger hits the bottom of the knee joint is Lv 7. Continue this line, and just above the knee you'll find Lv 8.

Once you have traced the meridian, go back over it and try to find any tight or sore spots. Release these using the release and dispersal pattern we've discussed. Also release the source point, Lv 3.

Key Points on the Liver Meridian

Lv 2   "Travel Between," for nausea, menstrual cramps, headaches.

Lv 3   "Great Thoroughfare," for headaches, vertigo, irritability, insomnia, toxicity, migraines.

Lv 4   "Draining Shells," for all reproductive disorders.

Lv 8   "Curved Spring," for menstrual problems, knee problems.

Lv 13   "Order Gate," for digestive problems, diarrhea. Spleen alarm point.

Lv 14   "Gate of Hope," the liver alarm point for chest tightness and rib pain, liver alarm and pancreas problems, vomiting into throat.

In addition to the key points on the meridian, you can also use the alarm point to disperse excessive energy and the Shu point to boost energy to the organ.

THE LIVER ALARM POINT

The alarm point (Lv 14) on the liver meridian can be used to diagnose the degree of imbalance in the organ and meridian. It is usually sensitive, but when it is acutely sensitive, it indicates that the organ is especially imbalanced and therefore the body is sending out a signal, or "alarm." An extremely painful alarm point usually indicates an excess of energy in the meridian, and that the condition is acute. A dull pain experienced when the alarm point is palpated indicates a more chronic condition. (See chapter 26 for more diagnostic details.) The point may also be swollen, a sign of chronic or long-standing problems within the liver; the organ itself is likely swollen, as well.

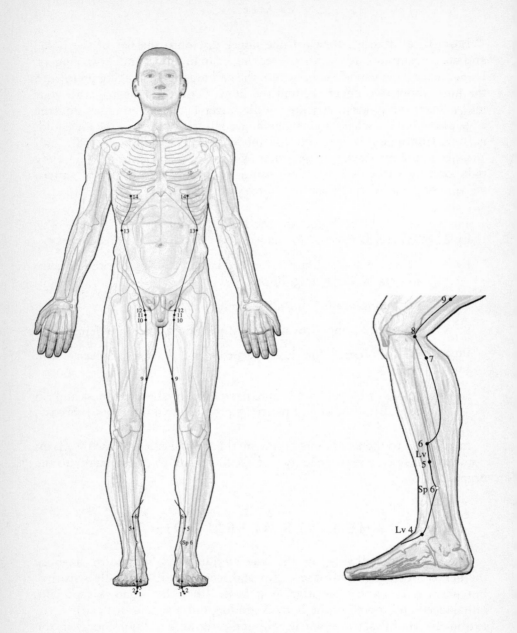

THE LIVER MERIDIAN

The alarm point of the liver meridian is found by starting at the bottom of the sternum, where a small bone, or "little tail," protrudes. This is called the xiphoid process (pronounced "ziffoid"). Don't apply too much pressure to this sensitive point. Now, in a straight line proceeding from the xiphoid process, measure four fingers directly below the sternum. Remember, one finger-width is about the width of the last segment of your index finger.

From the fourth finger-length distance, move laterally, about five fingers' distance, toward the left and right, as though you were measuring a band that ran along the chest, four fingers below the sternum. You will now be on the rib cage, in the space between the sixth and seventh ribs, known as the sixth intercostal space. Gently search with your hands for the sensitive point. This is Liver 14, the liver alarm point. It is the last point on the liver meridian.

THE LIVER SHU POINT

As we discussed in chapter 4, the Shu points are located along the spine and may be used for both diagnosis and treatment. Extremely sensitive Shu points indicate a general deficiency of Qi in the meridian and the related organ. If the liver Shu point is acutely sensitive or painful, disperse the Qi gently using a circular motion. If it is harder and more chronically congested, apply a gentle but deeper pressure to clear the congestion and send Qi into the meridian.

If you are working on yourself, you can stimulate the liver Shu points by putting two tennis balls into a sock, placing the balls and sock on the floor, and rolling your back on top of them along the spine.

The liver Shu point is located in the mid back area, just below the bottom of the shoulder blade (scapula). Find the bottom of the shoulder blade and trace a line from there straight across to the spine. You should be on a bone, the spinous process of the seventh thoracic vertebra. The spinous process is like a tail on the back of the vertebra; the tip is even with the bottom of the vertebra. Go down to the space between the spinous process to the eighth thoracic vertebra. The liver Shu point is found by dropping down to the next space between the eighth and ninth thoracic vertebrae and going out two fingers' distance.

Check to see if there is any apparent inflammation or tension here. Remember, if the tension is long-term, it will cover the whole area. Feel for a sense of fullness, which prevents you from determining with your fingers any of the details within the layers, such as muscle fibers, bones, or small points.

As you release this area, occasionally massage gently but deeply down the back, and on the back of the legs, along the bladder meridian. Concentrate your energy and focus in the area behind the knee, on Bl 40, which is very effective at releasing the back.

To find the point, bend the knee and put your thumb or finger into the depression directly behind the knee. Then straighten the knee; you will find that your finger is on a small mound directly behind the joint. Make sure that you are exactly in the middle of the back of the knee; that's where the point is located.

Gall Bladder Meridian

The gall bladder is a little pouch under the liver that holds bile acids and cholesterol. Bile acids emulsify and assist in the digestion of the fats we eat; at the same time, they keep the cholesterol within the gall bladder from forming stones. For its part, cholesterol buffers the bile acids and keeps them from irritating the organ. Together, the two work in perfect harmony—that is, until one or the other becomes imbalanced. Because of our love of high-fat foods, the gall bladder can easily be overwhelmed by fats and cholesterol. When that happens, the bile acids can no longer keep the cholesterol in check. The consequence is that the cholesterol forms crystals and then stones, which is the reason why so many gall bladders have to be surgically removed each year.

By following the guidelines offered below, you can clear the meridian and boost the flow of Qi, or life force, to the gall bladder, thereby strengthening and healing the organ.

The following physical and emotional symptoms indicate disharmonies in the gall bladder and gall bladder meridian.

Common Physical Symptoms of Imbalance

Headaches in temple (including migraines)

Ear and eye pain (especially outer corner of eye)

Joint stiffness and pain

Tightness or pain in sides of chest (ribs)

Nausea and vomiting

Yellow color in eyes

Stiffness in fourth toe

Gall stones

Common Emotional Symptoms of Imbalance
Anger, frustration (excess Qi)

Depression, lack of will (deficient Qi)

THE GALL BLADDER: FROM WEST AND EAST

The gall bladder is essentially a muscular pouch attached to the liver by a tube called the common duct. It is designed to hold bile acids and cholesterol, both produced by the liver. Bile acids are produced by the liver in order to break up or emulsify dietary fat.

In Chinese medicine, the gall bladder holds a much loftier place in the hierarchy of the human organs. Known traditionally as the "upright official who excels through his decisions and judgment," the gall bladder is said to play an essential role in a person's ability to make sound decisions. Good judgment and clear thinking are made possible, say the Chinese, when the gall bladder is balanced. When the organ is in disharmony, however, anger and frustration dominate and decision-making is clouded.

The gall bladder is also seen as an external manifestation of the liver energy. Thus, liver symptoms and signs become more pronounced when the gall bladder is imbalanced. Anger, for example, a symptom of liver imbalance, can become explosive and verbal, and illnesses related to both the liver and the gall bladder will be acute and inflamed.

When the liver energy becomes excessive, it can harm the gall bladder by producing excess bile, which irritates the gall bladder and digestive system. Especially sensitive to excess bile acids and fats is the duodenum, the first stage of the small intestine, where many ulcers form.

FINDING AND TREATING THE GALL BLADDER MERIDIAN

The first thing people tend to notice about the gall bladder meridian (GB) is that it zigzags back and forth over the head, and it zigzags down both sides of the body. The meridian begins at the outside corner of each eye, loops around the ear to the neck, goes back over the head to the forehead above the eyes, then over the head again to the back of the neck. From there, it drops down the neck and over the front of each shoulder. The meridian then zigzags down the sides of the body, along the outside of each leg, over the front of the ankles, and ends at the fourth toe. It is one of the longest meridians and provides Qi for both sides of the body.

When working on the gall bladder meridian, we are addressing both acute (short-term) obstructions to the flow of Qi and chronic (long-term) blockages that reflect a deep, internal imbalance. Points in an acute condition are more tender and sensitive and will announce themselves—either as pain or heat or as inflammation—almost immediately upon your touch. Points that have been blocked chronically can be more difficult to find, but in any case exist below layers of tension and congestion. (See chapter 4 for a fuller explanation of acute and chronic conditions.)

Remember, as you work gently with either acute or chronic points, you are using yin and yang to disperse areas that are excessive and to build up areas that are deficient.

RELEASING THE GALL BLADDER MERIDIAN

Begin by tracing the meridian. Then, as described in chapters 3 and 4, you will "release" the meridian by applying moderate pressure on the sensitive point until the tension dissipates and the energy flows from the point once again.

Let's begin the work of releasing the gall bladder meridian by treating the last point on the meridian, GB 44, which is found on the lateral (outside) base of the nail on the fourth toe. Gently massage the point and move up the toe until you are at the base of the fourth and fifth toes, at the webbing, pressing into the fourth metatarsal (the bone leading away from the fourth toe). From here, massage along the outside edge of the fourth metatarsal, moving toward the ankle while keeping your finger between the bones. Just before your fingers slide up onto the tarsal bones you'll find GB 41. Spend a minute gently releasing this point.

Continue massaging toward the ankle; here you will find a depression about the size of the tip of your thumb, just in front of and a little below the lateral malleolus (the outside bump on your ankle). This is GB 40, the source point for the gall bladder meridian. Experiment with different ways to massage this point; it should be somewhat tender.

From here, massage up the leg just in front of the lateral malleolus and onto the fibula bone, on the outside of the leg. Massage up the fibula to halfway between the lateral malleolus and the side of the knee, then drop back just behind the fibula. Feel for a sensitive point found in a very small depression; this is GB 35. From here, massage up while moving toward the front of the fibula, at the knee.

The top of the fibula is a big bump. Just in front of that bump is GB 34, a point that boosts both vitality and resistance to disease. It will very likely be sensitive, giving the client a mild electric sensation. End by massaging up over the knee joint to GB 33, just behind the tendon that attaches on the side of the knee.

Once you have traced the meridian, go back over it and find any tight or particularly sensitive points. Release these using the release and dispersal pattern. Also release the source point again.

Key Points on the Gall Bladder Meridian

GB 34   "Yang Mound Spring," for sprains, pains, joint stiffness, stomach cramps, constipation.

GB 37   "Bright Light," for all eye problems.

GB 39   "Suspended Bell," for headaches (usually acts within ten seconds), hearing disorders (tinnitus, gradual hearing loss).

GB 40   "Hill's Ruins," for knee, hip, lower back, and rib pain; neck stiffness. Gall bladder source point.

GB 41   "Foot Verge of Tears," for vision and eye problems, menstrual disorders.

In addition to the points described above, you can also use the alarm point to disperse excessive energy and the Shu point to boost deficient energy to the organ.

THE GALL BLADDER ALARM POINT

The alarm point for the gall bladder, GB 24, is on the front of the rib cage, down from the sternum. It is directly below Liver 14, in the next

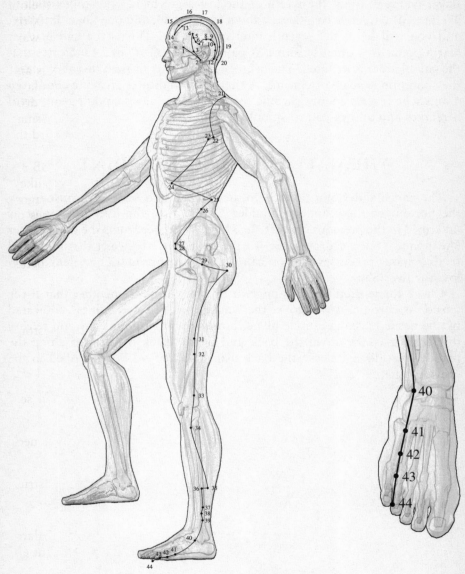

THE GALL BLADDER MERIDIAN

intercostal space between the ribs in the front of the body. To find Liver 14, move four fingers down from the base of the sternum (toward your feet), and five fingers laterally (to the sides of the body) until you are between the sixth and seventh ribs, known as the sixth intercostal space. (One finger-width is about the width of the last segment of your index finger.) To find GB 24, move two fingers down from Lv 14, and one finger laterally, and you will be at the seventh intercostal space. This is the gall bladder alarm point. It is often sensitive. A painful or swollen GB 24 indicates that the gall bladder is irritated. The degree of sensitivity or pain reveals whether the condition is acute or chronic. A sharp pain indicates an acute condition; a dull ache reveals a more chronic condition. Massage the point gently until it relaxes and allows you to stimulate it.

THE GALL BLADDER SHU POINT

The gall bladder Shu point is located in the mid back area, just below the bottom of the scapula (shoulder blade). Find the liver Shu point as described in the previous chapter. Just below the liver Shu is the gall bladder Shu point. You can drop down to the next space between the ninth and tenth spinous processes, or you can simply measure two finger-lengths below the liver Shu.

Check for tension or any apparent inflammation. Remember that if the tension is chronic, it will cover the whole area. Feel for fullness, indicated by the tissue masking muscle fibers, bones, or small points. As you release this area, massage down the back and on the back of the legs along the bladder meridian. Release the back using Bladder 40 (as described in the previous chapter).

Spleen Meridian

In Chinese medicine, the spleen is seen as the governor of digestion and the very core of the immune system. Therefore, it is among the most important of all your organs. By clearing the spleen meridian, you will enhance the function of your entire digestive tract and help overcome all forms of indigestion, including dyspepsia, diarrhea, and constipation. By simply following the instructions you will boost the flow of Qi to both the spleen and the spleen meridian, and thereby enhance the health of the organ and assist in it overcoming any existing disorders.

The following physical and emotional symptoms indicate disharmonies in the spleen and spleen meridian.

Common Physical Symptoms of Imbalance

Heartburn, acid indigestion, and nausea

Belching and gas

Digestive problems (including constipation or diarrhea)

Immune deficiency or disorders

Lymphatic problems (swollen lymph nodes)

Hypoglycemia or diabetes

Abdominal distention

Appetite imbalance

Heavy, aching body

Knee or thigh problems

Memory problems

Vomiting after eating

Common Emotional Symptoms of Imbalance
Excessive worry (excess Qi)

Sensitivity (excess Qi)

Obsession, "tunnel vision" (deficient Qi)

Lack of awareness (deficient Qi)

THE SPLEEN: FROM WEST AND EAST

The spleen is located within the left part of the abdomen, under the left rib cage. It is a soft, blood-filled organ, capable of expansion and contraction, and thereby taking up or releasing blood into general circulation. In this way, the spleen helps to regulate how much blood is in circulation, thus meeting the body's needs for oxygen. Exercise causes the spleen to contract and release blood; resting causes the spleen to expand and take up blood.

Western medicine regards the spleen, as it does the gall bladder, as essentially an expendable organ. When the spleen is removed, the liver and lymph system are thought to assume its functions, though it is known that the immune system is weakened with the loss of the spleen.

The spleen performs three functions, according to Western medicine. The first is to introduce immune cells into the blood as blood passes through the organ. Second, the spleen filters the blood and cleanses it of broken blood vessels, debris from red cells, and bacteria. Third, it acts as a reservoir of blood, releasing extra blood when needed.

From the Western perspective, the spleen is part of the lymphatic system, a vast network of vessels, ducts, and trunks, not unlike our circulatory system, only without a central pump, or heart. The lymph system moves fluids and toxins from the cells to the blood, which brings these constituents to the liver for detoxification. The lymph system also absorbs fats from the digestive system and brings them to the blood.

In Chinese medicine, the spleen is linked with the pancreas, which creates digestive enzymes that break down carbohydrates and proteins and which balances the blood sugar level through the production of the hormone insulin.

Traditional Chinese medicine sees the spleen as having a much more important role. The spleen is regarded as the primary organ of digestion, passing Qi to the small and large intestines. Whether the spleen passes on chaotic or harmonious Qi to these organs determines the capacity of the small intestine to assimilate nutrients and the large intestine to eliminate waste. The spleen is highly sensitive to excessive consumption of sugar and acidic foods. When the spleen is weakened by such foods, it is unable to pass sufficient energy on to the intestines, often resulting in chronic indigestion and constipation.

During digestion, the spleen provides the Qi needed to separate the "pure" from the "impure," meaning those constituents in our food that we require for health, versus those we should eliminate.

The Chinese also credit the spleen with maintaining the elasticity of blood vessels, thereby sustaining diastolic pressure throughout the system. Proper circulation is dependent on a healthy spleen, which keeps the blood in its channels and provides Qi to the blood and its vessels. Therefore the spleen, as well as the heart, would be treated when curing circulation problems. Conditions such as hemorrhoids, varicose veins, aneurysms, internal bleeding, and strokes are all related to the health of the spleen.

FINDING AND TREATING THE SPLEEN MERIDIAN

The spleen meridian (Sp) begins at the inside of the big toe, at the nail, runs along the inside of the foot, turns upward in front of the ankle bone, then ascends along the inside of the calf, to the knee. From there the meridian runs up through the genital region, through the abdomen and to the spleen itself, and then to the stomach. The meridian continues upward, along the side of the body and chest area to the outside of the breast.

When working on the spleen meridian, we are addressing both acute (short-term) obstructions to the flow of Qi and chronic (long-term) blockages that reflect a deep, internal imbalance. Points in an acute condition are more tender and sensitive and will announce themselves—either as pain or heat or as inflammation—almost immediately upon your touch. Points that have been blocked chronically can be more difficult to find, but in any case exist below layers of tension and congestion. (See chapter 4 for a fuller explanation of acute and chronic conditions.)

Remember, as you work gently with either acute or chronic points, you are using yin and yang to disperse areas that are excessive and to build up areas that are deficient.

RELEASING THE SPLEEN MERIDIAN

Begin by tracing the meridian. Then, as described in chapters 3 and 4, you will "release" the meridian by applying moderate pressure on each of the sensitive points until the tension dissipates and the energy flows from the point once again.

Stimulate the meridian in general, beginning at Sp 1, located at the medial side of the big toe, at the base of the nail. Massage proximally (toward the ankle) along the line where the top and side of the big toe meet, until you come to the base knuckle. Just before the base knuckle is Sp 2, and just beyond that is Sp 3, the source or balancing point. It is located in the niche formed by the back of the base knuckle where it meets the underside of the first metatarsal.

From there, slide along under the first metatarsal two finger-lengths. One finger-length is about the width of the last segment of your index finger. You will feel a bump in the bone as you reach the posterior end of the first metatarsal. Spleen 4 is located where the shaft of the bone meets the bump. Slide back and somewhat up to the ankle just in front of the medial malleolus (the inside ankle bump), to Sp 5.

Spleen 6 is a very important point. It is the meeting point of the three yin meridians of the legs—spleen, liver, and kidney. It is often used to treat reproductive problems and is incorporated into many other treatment patterns. It is located five fingers above the medial malleolus, the big bump on the inside of the ankle joint. Find the center of the medial malleolus (the peak) and put your little finger on it and put the other fingers against the bone (the tibia) so that the index finger is the closest to the knee, with each finger barely touching the next finger. This is three fingers' distance—as I said before, even though you have four fingers touching, we don't count the first finger.

You need to measure two more fingers, which you can do with the other hand. Put the middle finger of the other hand above the index finger, and the other index finger above that and you have measured five fingers—to Sp 6, on the edge of the bone. It will be somewhat sore and feel like a little niche in the sharp edge of the bone.

From here, the meridian runs up just behind the tibia to the knee. Four fingers above Sp 6 is Sp 7. Spleen 8 is five fingers up from Sp 7, and Sp 9 is located four fingers above Sp 8. Spleen 9 is in the niche formed by the shaft of the tibia where it widens into the knee joint, pressing behind the

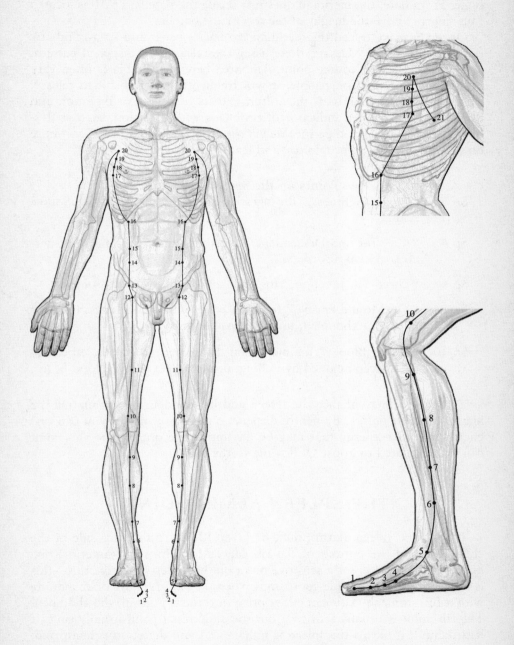

THE SPLEEN MERIDIAN

bone. From here, the meridian goes just inside the patella; Sp 10 is located four fingers above the height of the top of the patella.

Once you have traced the meridian, go back over it and try to find any tight or sore spots. Massage these using the release and dispersal pattern, and also release the source point. The area behind the tibia is often very bumpy and stagnant on people; it will frequently feel difficult to release. This reflects problems with the spleen and its functions of digestion and immunity. It is a good indicator of problems with digestion, such as dysbiosis (bad bacteria) and permeable gut syndrome. (See chapter 27 for more on intestinal bacteria, probiotics, and leaky gut syndrome.)

Key Points on the Spleen Meridian

Sp 3   "Great Brightness," for digestive problems, poor appetite. Source point.

Sp 4   "Ancestor and Descendent," for abdominal pain, diarrhea, nervous system disorders.

Sp 6   "Three Yin Junction," for male and female sexual problems.

Sp 9   "Yin Mound Spring," for knee pain; pain and coldness in lower back and abdomen; urinary dysfunctions.

Sp 10   "Sea of Blood," for menstrual disorders; red rashes, especially those accompanied by itching; dispersing excessive blood heat.

You can further enhance the spleen and its meridian by stimulating the alarm and Shu points. By gently dispersing the alarm point, you can discharge excessive energy that may be disrupting the organ. The Shu point can be stimulated to boost Qi flowing to the organ.

THE SPLEEN ALARM POINT

To find the spleen alarm point, or Liver 13, go to the very side of the chest and find the bottom of the rib cage. Move forward (anterior) one finger-width and feel for a sensitive point on the underside of the ribs—this is typically the area people get cramps when they are running or swimming with a full stomach. You can either press into the rib or into the abdomen. The rib point is usually sensitive, but the abdominal point usually isn't. If it is painful, it means the spleen is imbalanced and digestion is hampered. Gently disperse this point.

THE SPLEEN SHU POINT

Your own Shu points, on Bladder 20, can only be reached with a partner, or by putting two tennis balls in a sock, placing them on the floor, and then rolling your back over the balls.

The spleen Shu point is located outside the eleventh and twelfth thoracic vertebrae, just above the bottom of the rib cage. Find the very bottom of the ribs at the side of the back, and trace a line from there straight across to the spine. You should be on the spinous process of the second lumbar vertebra. The spinous process is like a tail on the back of the vertebra; the tip is even with the bottom of the vertebra.

The spleen Shu point is located two fingers above the bottom rib, and two fingers outside the spinous process of thoracic 11.

Stimulate deeply, noticing if one side is fuller than the other and working more on that side. As you release this area, you should occasionally massage down the back and on the back of the legs along the bladder meridian. Spend extra time in the area behind the knee as there is a point here, Bl 40, which is very helpful in releasing the back. To find the point, bend the knee and put your thumb or finger into the depression behind the knee. When you straighten the knee, you will find that you are actually on a small mound, directly behind the joint. Make sure that you are exactly in the middle of the back of the knee. Stimulate this point gently, but deeply.

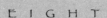

Stomach Meridian

We experience such misery when the stomach isn't working properly. The stomach prepares food for digestion and, by doing so, enhances the function of the small and large intestines.

By clearing the stomach and stomach meridian, you will enhance the health and function of not only the organ, but your entire digestive system. You will improve your assimilation of nutrients and your ability to eliminate waste. Simply follow the guidelines offered below and, within minutes, you can clear the meridian and boost the flow of Qi, or life force, to the stomach, the stomach meridian, and the small and large intestines.

The following physical and emotional symptoms indicate disharmonies in the stomach and stomach meridian.

Common Physical Symptoms of Imbalance

Abdomen (upper) distention

Groaning

Yawning

Jaw tension

Knee pain or swelling

Lip or mouth sores

Mouth sideways, crooked

Neck or throat swollen

Vomiting

Abdomen swollen, full

Cold in stomach area

Frequent hunger or thirst

Sleepy after eating

Abdominal pain

Common Emotional Symptoms of Imbalance

Critical

Lack of understanding

Lack of compassion

Anxiety, chronic nervous tension

Inability to feel emotionally stable, centered

THE STOMACH: FROM WEST AND EAST

Shaped like a boxing glove, the stomach is a muscular sac joined to the esophagus at the top and to the small intestine at the bottom. Western medicine holds that the stomach has five functions: storing food; making digestive juices; churning the food into a homogenous mix called chyme; digesting proteins from foods; and releasing the treated food into the small intestine.

In Chinese medicine it is said that the stomach takes the gross matter of the food and passes the pure essence, or energy, on to the spleen. The Chinese saw the stomach and spleen as intimately connected, each one providing Qi to the other. Thus, the stomach and spleen are regarded as paired organs, often referred to in Chinese medicine as the yang and yin organs of the Earth Element, in the Five Element system. (See chapter 25, "The Five Elements.") Together, the stomach and spleen control digestion by dispersing Qi throughout the digestive tract.

Since the stomach meridian begins at the mouth, it is said to control the mouth, tongue, and esophagus. Thus, it nourishes and controls the preparation of food for digestion.

One notable difference between the Western and Eastern views of the stomach is that in Chinese medicine, which is more concerned with function, the duodenum is considered to be part of the stomach, whereas in Western physiology the duodenum is considered to be the first part of the small intestine. Functionally, the duodenum is where the pancreas and liver both secrete their digestive juices; it is an area, therefore, more related to preparation of food than to assimilation.

FINDING AND TREATING THE STOMACH MERIDIAN

Starting below the eyes, the stomach meridian (St) descends to the sides of the mouth and the jaw, from which a branch rises to the forehead. It continues along the side of the throat to the collarbone and over the chest and abdomen to the pubic area. From there, it passes along the front of the thigh to the outside of the kneecap. Below the kneecap, the meridian divides into two branches, one of which ends at the second toe and the other at the third toe.

When working on the stomach meridian, we are addressing both acute (short-term) obstructions to the flow of Qi and chronic (long-term) blockages that reflect a deep, internal imbalance. Points in an acute condition are more tender and sensitive and will announce themselves—either as pain or heat or as inflammation—almost immediately upon your touch. Points that have been blocked chronically can be more difficult to find, but in any case exist below layers of tension and congestion. (See chapter 4 for a fuller explanation of acute and chronic conditions.)

Remember, as you work gently with either acute or chronic points, you are using yin and yang to disperse areas that are excessive and to build up areas that are deficient.

RELEASING THE STOMACH MERIDIAN

Begin by tracing the meridian. Then, as described in chapters 3 and 4, you will "release" the meridian by applying moderate pressure on each of the sensitive points until the tension dissipates and the energy flows from the point once again.

There are actually two paths of the stomach meridian from the knee down. Most meridian charts simply show a path running from just below the outside of the patella (kneecap) and making a zigzag in the middle of the shin, then continuing on to the second toe. Actually, the meridian splits at St 36, just below the patella, and the two parts follow parallel courses to the second and third toes. For the stomach meridian, St 40 is the only generally recognized point on the outer branch meridian, but as we will see it is an important one.

Start by massaging the meridian from its end point at the lateral (outside) base of the nail on the second toe. This is St 45. Massage up the toe until you are between the base knuckles of the second and third toes, at the webbing, pressing into the second toe (St 44). From here, go just past the knuckle and massage against the second metatarsal where it meets the knuckle (St 43). Massage along the outside edge of the second metatarsal, moving toward the ankle while keeping your finger between the bones. A little less than halfway to the ankle, you will reach the tarsal bones. Just before your finger slides up onto the tarsal bones is St 42, which is the source, or balancing, point for the stomach meridian.

Continue massaging toward the ankle; just at the ankle, in a depression just to the outside of a bundle of tendons, is St 41. From here, you want to move halfway between the ankle and the knee joint, just below the patella (kneecap) and just outside the tibia. To do this, place the tip of the ring finger of your right hand on the ankle just outside St 41 and the thumb of your left hand on the knee joint just below and outside the patella. Stretch the left ring finger toward the ankle and the right thumb toward the knee, touching them together. Make sure both hands are stretching the same amount, and that they meet halfway up the shin.

Just outside the tibia in the belly of the anterior tibialis muscle is St 38, and just two fingers out from there is St 40, which is a great point for draining excess mucus from the upper body, i.e., the lungs and sinuses. Stomach 39 is located just two fingers below St 38. Stomach 38 and St 39 are located on the inner branch of the stomach meridian, and St 40 is located on the outer branch.

From here, massage up the inner branch to St 37, located three fingers above St 38. Five fingers above that is St 36, perhaps the most revered point in acupuncture because of its unparalleled ability to increase the energy of the body. This point is routinely stimulated very strongly by athletes in the days and hours before an important event to increase endurance and stamina. In some schools of acupuncture there are up to four alternate locations for St 36, so you should try to stimulate the entire area of the upper anterior tibialis muscle.

Find where the tibia bone widens just before the knee joint and put the tips of the fingers of your opposite hand into the muscle just below, with the palm against the other side of the tibia for leverage. Take the same side hand and use it to press the fingers in deeper, and then roll your fingers deeply across the muscle. You should feel a deep ache and possibly have some sensation down into the lower leg and toes (this is called "getting Qi"). It will usually continue to ache after you release.

From here, the meridian passes over the knee just outside the patella. Stomach 35 is located at the joint, even with the bottom of the patella, and St 34 is located four fingers above the height of the top of the patella.

Spend some time massaging the meridian, especially down both branches. Find any tight or sore spots. Release these using the release and dispersal pattern we covered earlier and also release the source point again. Look for areas of fullness and congestion and try to move this "stuck Qi" down through the meridian. Try moving it upward as well, and see the difference. Often, it is easier to "unlock" the meridian by releasing against its direction of flow.

Key Points on the Stomach Meridian

St 36   "Foot Three Miles," for strength and endurance, all digestive and intestinal disorders, all deficiency disorders, lung disorders, immunity, gall and kidney stones, knee problems.

St 40   "Abundant Flourishing," for excess mucus, lung disorders, anxiety and insomnia, sore throat, dizziness.

St 42   "Rushing Yang," for lack of appetite, digestive problems, tooth and mouth problems. Stomach source point.

St 45   "Evil's Dissipation," for calming and uplifting the spirit.

In addition to the points I mentioned on the stomach meridian, you can also stimulate the alarm and Shu points. Stimulating the alarm point can disperse excessive energy trapped in the stomach, and stimulating the Shu point can boost deficient energy in the organ.

THE STOMACH ALARM POINT

Begin your treatment of the stomach meridian by stimulating the stomach alarm point, which is found at the front of the body, right below the sternum. To find the point, go to the very bottom of the sternum, or breastbone. There, you will find a small bone, called the xiphoid process (pronounced "ziffoid"). This is a sensitive area, so avoid applying too much pressure. From the xiphoid process, measure five finger-lengths downward, toward the navel. One finger length is roughly the width of the last segment of your index finger. Gently probe this area for a tender, electric energetic well, which is Conception Vessel 12, or the stomach alarm point. If the point is sensitive to the touch, or painful, the stomach is irritated or in disharmony. Disperse the point gently to allow excessive energy to be discharged and the stomach and stomach meridian to be harmonized.

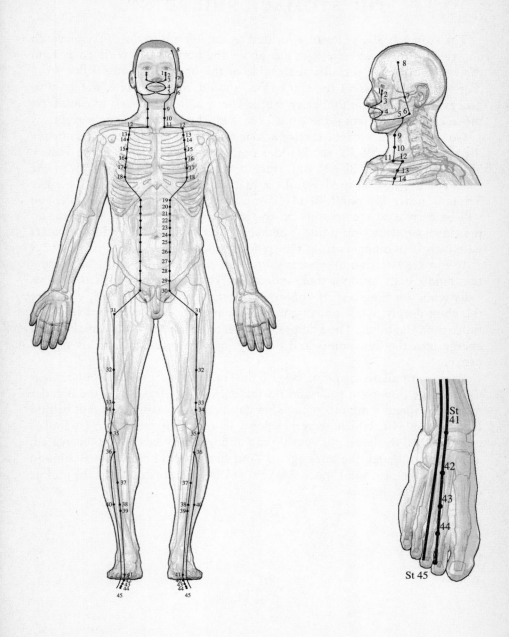

THE STOMACH MERIDIAN

THE STOMACH SHU POINT

The stomach Shu points are located to the left and right of the eleventh and twelfth thoracic vertebrae, just above the bottom of the rib cage. Find the very bottom of the ribs at the side of the back, and trace a line from there straight across to the spine. You should be on a bone, the spinous process of the second lumbar vertebra. The spinous process is like a tail on the back of the vertebra; the tip is even with the bottom of the vertebra.

Go to the outside of the erector spinae muscles, about four fingers outside the spine (this is Bl 52, the bladder point located just outside the kidney Shu point, which is Bl 23), and trace up until you feel the bottom of the ribs. You are now at the level of the first lumbar vertebra (this is the outer Triple Warmer Shu point, Bl 51). If you move up two fingers' distance, you will be even with the spinous process of the twelfth thoracic vertebra, on the outer stomach Shu point. The actual Shu point is located two fingers in, which is two fingers from the spinous process.

If you are working on yourself, you can stimulate this point by placing two tennis balls inside a sock and rolling your back on top of the tennis balls while on the floor. If you are working with someone else, stimulate the point deeply, while noticing if one side is more swollen, or inflamed, or fuller than the other. The Shu points indicate deficiency. You can also send energy into the Shu points and directly into the meridian and its related organ.

As you stimulate the point, release the entire area around the point. Gently massage down the back and on the back of the legs along the bladder meridian. Spend a minute gently stimulating and releasing the point behind the knee, Bl 40, which is very helpful in releasing the back. To find it exactly, bend the knee, put your thumb or finger into the depression created, and then straighten the knee again. Your fingers will be on a small mound directly behind the joint space. Make sure that you are exactly in the middle of the back of the knee.

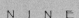

Heart Meridian

As the old song says, "You've got to have heart," and in Chinese medicine, we mean that in more ways than one. From the Eastern point of view, the heart is the home of the spirit, meaning your awareness of yourself and your environment. In the West, the most troubled organ is the heart. More people die of illnesses related to the heart and circulatory system than of any other cause. At the same time, the quality of our lives depends on the extent to which we know and understand our own hearts. In both the physical and the metaphorical senses, there is no more profound and essential part of each of us than the human heart.

In this chapter, I will show you how to clear the heart meridian, and thereby restore Qi, or life force, to the heart, which will help the heart and its meridian to overcome existing cardiovascular disorders.

The following physical and emotional symptoms indicate disharmonies in the heart and heart meridian.

Common Physical Symptoms of Imbalance

Hot or cold hands and feet

Nervousness, irritability

Red complexion

Mental or emotional disturbance

Insomnia, disturbed sleep, or excessive dreaming

Cardiovascular disorders

Brain or nervous system disorders

Speech problems

Spontaneous sweating

Poor memory of important life events

Common Emotional Symptoms of Imbalance

Excessive laughter (excess Qi)

Hysteria (excess Qi)

Expressionless appearance (deficient Qi)

Lack of joy (deficient Qi)

THE HEART: FROM WEST AND EAST

The heart, located behind the sternum, is actually two pumps, each one perfectly coordinated with the other. The left side of the heart serves as a pump for the general circulation, pumping oxygen-rich blood to every cell in the body. The right side pumps venous blood, carrying carbon dioxide to the lungs. Because the job of pumping blood to the general circulation is much more difficult—there's a lot more resistance and a lot more distance to travel—the left side of the heart is more muscular, stronger, and larger. On average, the heart beats sixty to eighty times per minute, cycling the entire blood supply of the body through the heart in sixty seconds.

In Chinese medicine, the heart is regarded as the "palace of the Shen" (Shen being the human spirit). The Shen is the source of our consciousness, that aspect of ourselves that defines our identity, makes us self-aware, and also keeps us conscious of our interdependence with others. It is also the source of our vitality, especially when the Shen is directed toward something it loves. (For more on the Chinese understanding of the heart, see chapter 25, "The Five Elements.")

In its role as the center of emotional and mental consciousness, the heart meridian rules both the heart and the mind. It is associated with passion, mental clarity, and joy. By controlling the blood flow to the brain, the heart also is seen to regulate memory and other brain functions.

FINDING AND TREATING THE HEART MERIDIAN

The heart meridian (Ht) begins at the heart and surfaces in the center of the armpit. The meridian passes down the inside of the arm, crosses the inner point of the elbow fold, and runs through to the tip of the little finger. It terminates at a point on the thumb-side of the pinky nail.

When working on the heart meridian, we are addressing both acute (short-term) obstructions to the flow of Qi and chronic (long-term) blockages that reflect a deep, internal imbalance. Points in an acute condition are more tender and sensitive and will announce themselves—either as pain or heat or as inflammation—almost immediately upon your touch. Points that have been blocked chronically can be more difficult to find, but in any case exist below layers of tension and congestion.

Remember, as you work gently with either acute or chronic points, you are using yin and yang to disperse areas that are excessive and to build up areas that are deficient.

RELEASING THE HEART MERIDIAN

Begin by tracing the meridian. Then, as described in chapters 3 and 4, you will "release" the meridian by applying moderate pressure on all the sensitive points until the tension dissipates and the energy flows from the point once again.

Clearing the heart meridian promotes circulation and profound calm. To begin, massage the meridian starting at the inside of the little finger at the base of the nail—this is Ht 9. Massage along the inside of the little finger until you come to the webbed area between the metacarpal bones. Here, move on to the palm side in a direct line toward the pisiform, the bump at the wrist (located on the medial, or pinky-side of the hand where it meets the wrist and the ulna, one of the two bones of the forearm).

Just past the pisiform at the underside of the wrist joint is Ht 7, the source point. The point is on the underside of the wrist, within the crease of the wrist, on a line with the pinky. Press firmly and find this sensitive point.

As you move up the arm from Ht 7, you'll find three other points along the tendon—in a row, each less than a finger apart from each other. These are Ht 6, Ht 5, and Ht 4. Massage each of these points gently, firmly, and deeply. All the work you do on the heart meridian should be done gently. The motion is a kind of gentle rubbing massage, dispersing the energy trapped within the meridian.

Keep massaging along the medial (pinky-side) forearm until you get to the elbow. With the palm faceup, find the crease of the inner elbow joint and go to the medial (pinky-)side. Heart 3 is a wide finger-width distance, moving into the crease from the "funny bone" bump. This point reflects the quality of the nervous system and heart—if it is tight and knotted, the person is high-strung and tense. If it is full and congested, there may be some form of congestion within the cardiovascular system.

From here, the meridian goes up the inside of the arm. A little less than halfway between the elbow and the armpit on the inside of the humerus is Ht 2. This point called the *joie de vivre* (joy of life) point in French acupuncture, is very helpful in treating depression or sadness. The meridian goes on to the center of the armpit, where we find Ht 1. Massage deeply.

Once you have traced the meridian, go back over it and try to find any tight or sore spots. Release these using the release and dispersal pattern discussed earlier, and also release the source point.

Key Points on the Heart Meridian

Ht 2   "Green Spring," for depression and sorrow. The *joie de vivre* (joy of life) point in French acupuncture.

Ht 3   "Lesser Sea," for calming the spirit; forgetfulness and disorientation; chest pain; sudden loss of voice.

Ht 5   "Communication's Route," for clear thinking, calming the spirit.

Ht 7   "Spirit's Gate," for calming the spirit, clear thinking, heart problems, throat and tongue problems.

Ht 8   "Lesser Palace," for calming the spirit (great for children); heart problems.

Ht 9   "Lesser Rushing," along with SI 1, for heart attack. Use very strong stimulation, usually to the left pinky finger.

You can also use the alarm point to disperse excessive energy and the Shu point to boost deficient energy to the organ.

THE HEART ALARM POINT

The heart alarm point is found on the front of the body, just below the sternum, and right above the stomach alarm point. Go to the bottom of the sternum, or breastbone, and find the little bone at the very bottom— the xiphoid process (discussed in previous chapters). Remember, the bone

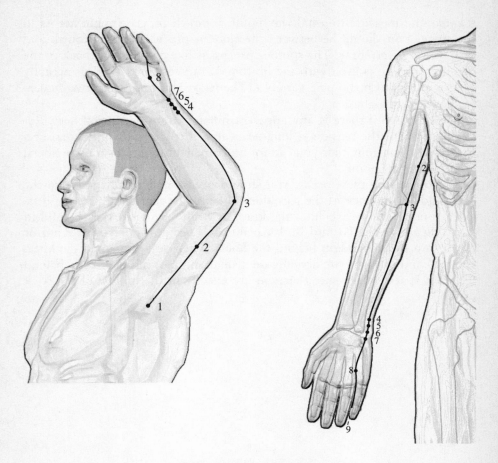

THE HEART MERIDIAN

is very sensitive; do not apply excessive pressure. Measure five fingers below the sternum and you will find Conception Vessel 15, the circulation/pericardium alarm point. One finger below that is the heart alarm point. Massage the point gently—it is often very sensitive—and disperse the energy emanating from it.

THE HEART SHU POINT

The heart Shu point is located in the upper back area, at the vertical middle of the scapulae (shoulder blades). Find the top and bottom of the scapula and measure to a halfway point. From there, go straight across to the spine. You should be between the spinous processes of the fourth and fifth thoracic vertebrae. The spinous process is like a tail on the back of the vertebra; the tip is even with the bottom of the vertebra. You are actually even with the fifth thoracic vertebra. The heart Shu points are two fingers to the left and right.

Check to see if there is any apparent inflammation or tension here. Remember that if the tension is long-term, it will cover the whole area. Feel for fullness, meaning that you cannot find any details such as muscle fibers, bones, or small points.

As you release these areas, you should occasionally massage down the back and on the back of the legs along the bladder meridian. Spend a little extra time in the area behind the knee, at Bl 40, which is very helpful in releasing the back. To find Bl 40, bend the knee and put your thumb or finger into the depression behind the knee. When you straighten the knee, you will find that you are actually on a small mound; this is directly behind the joint space. Make sure that you are exactly in the middle of the back of the knee.

Small Intestine Meridian

*Chinese medicine, in its typi-*cally poetic way, says that the small intestine is the official in charge of receiving, filling, and transforming. The Western perspective is not much different.

The small intestine is responsible for taking the nutrients from the foods you eat and assimilating them into the bloodstream, a task that is essential for life. You could be on the best diet in the world and still not get everything you need if your small intestine is not working correctly.

In this chapter, I'm going to show you how to clear the small intestine meridian and thereby support an organ that you depend on for life.

The following symptoms may arise when the small intestine and small intestine meridian are imbalanced.

Common Physical Symptoms of Imbalance

Lower abdomen distended

Arm pain (as if broken)

Cheeks swollen

Head difficult to turn to side

Shoulder pain, tension

Swellings or nodules between tendons

Elbow joint stiff or sore

Eyes sore or red

Disorders related to the small intestine (including Crohn's disease)

Common Emotional Symptoms of Imbalance
Lack of mental clarity or judgment (deficient Qi)

Lack of joy (deficient Qi)

Excessively emotional (excess Qi)

Hysteria (excess Qi)

THE SMALL INTESTINE: FROM WEST AND EAST

The small intestine is about an inch and a half in diameter and approximately twenty-two feet long. The organ tends to be about a foot longer in Asians, whose diets have been grain-centered for thousands of years, than in Westerners', whose diets have included large quantities of animal foods for the past one hundred years.

The small intestine consists of three parts: the duodenum, about ten inches long, which starts at the pyloric sphincter of the stomach and receives bile acids and pancreatic enzymes; next comes the eight-foot-long jejunum; then the last is the ileum, about twelve feet long, which ends at the cecum, the first section of the large intestine. At the junction of the ileum and the cecum is the ileocecal valve, which allows digested food (chyme) to move into the large intestine but does not allow backflow into the small intestine.

The small intestine's work of digesting and absorbing nutrients is assisted by the presence of trillions of bacteria, many of which aid in the breakdown of food particles. Food takes an average of five to six hours to pass through the small intestine.

According to Chinese medicine, imbalances in the small intestine prevent the smooth transfer of Qi from the food to the stomach and the spleen. This means that the separation of the pure and the impure—or the gross food matter from the pure energy, or life force—does not efficiently take place. The result is a depletion of life force within the digestive tract, a host of digestive disorders, and poor assimilation of nutrition.

In Chinese medicine, the small intestine is seen as linked with the heart, helping it to bring clarity of mind, distinguishing and assimilating good ideas.

FINDING AND TREATING THE SMALL INTESTINE MERIDIAN

The small intestine meridian (SI) begins at the outside of the nail on the little finger, trails the back of the hand to the wrist and follows the outside of the ulna to the elbow. It follows the back of the arm up to the shoulder joint, where it crosses the shoulder blade to the collarbone. From here, the meridian continues up the side of the neck and over the cheek to the ear.

When working on the small intestine meridian, we are addressing both acute (short-term) obstructions to the flow of Qi and chronic (long-term) blockages that reflect a deep, internal imbalance. Points in an acute condition will be more tender and sensitive and will announce themselves—either as pain or heat or as inflammation—almost immediately upon your touch. Points that have been blocked chronically can be more difficult to find, but in any case exist below layers of tension and congestion. (See chapter 4 for a fuller explanation of acute and chronic conditions.)

Remember, as you work gently with either acute or chronic points, you are using yin and yang to disperse areas that are excessive and to build up areas that are deficient.

RELEASING THE SMALL INTESTINE MERIDIAN

Begin by tracing the meridian. Then, as described in chapters 3 and 4, you will "release" the meridian by applying moderate pressure on each of the sensitive points until the tension dissipates and the energy flows from the point once again.

Start by massaging the meridian at SI 1, the point located at the lateral (outside) base of the nail on the little finger. Massage up the finger to the base knuckle of the little finger. From here, massage along the outside edge of the fifth metacarpal (the bone above the knuckle) to the wrist. A little more than halfway to the wrist, you will reach the bump at the end of the fifth metacarpal. Go just past the bump and you will feel a niche, a gap between the fifth metacarpal and the carpal bones. This is SI 4, the source point. Release this point to balance the entire meridian.

One finger up from SI 4 is the wrist and SI 5. Move toward the elbow two fingers and up onto the top of the ulna to SI 6. From here, the meridian goes back to the medial side of the arm. Massage just under the ulna up to the elbow. You are following the path of the ulnar nerve. At the elbow, you should be between two bumps, the medial epicondyle and the tip of the elbow, the olecranon process. This is where the "funny bone" is located;

it's actually the most vulnerable location of the ulnar nerve. It is also the location for SI 8.

Once you have traced the meridian, go back over it and try to find any tight or sore spots. Release these using the release and dispersal pattern we covered earlier, and also release the source point again.

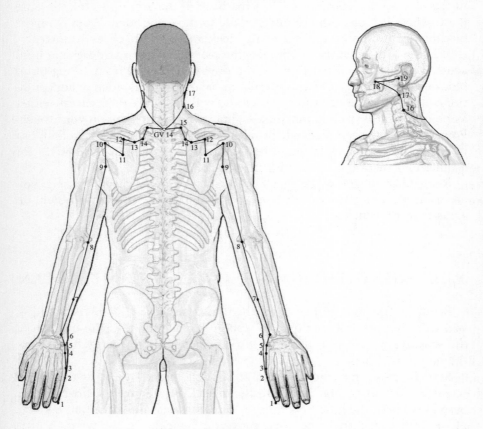

THE SMALL INTESTINE MERIDIAN

Key Points on the Small Intestine Meridian

SI 1   "Young Marsh," along with Ht 9, for heart attack. Use very strong stimulation and pressure, usually to the left pinky finger. Also, for loss of consciousness.

SI 3   "Black Stream," for strengthening the spine; relaxing the muscles; ear troubles.

SI 4   "Wrist Bone," for pain and stiffness of neck. Small intestine source point.

SI 6   "Supporting the Old," for loosening tight neck, shoulders, and lower back; any existing eye problems.

SI 10   "Scapula's Hollow," the shoulder release point.

In addition to clearing the meridian, you can also use the alarm point to disperse excess energy within the meridian, and the Shu point to boost energy to the organ itself.

THE SMALL INTESTINE ALARM POINT

The small intestine alarm point is just above the pubic bone, about five fingers' distance toward the navel. This is Conception Vessel 4. If it feels sensitive with deep pressure, it indicates that the small intestine is irritated or imbalanced. Massage gently and disperse the energy emanating from it.

THE SMALL INTESTINE SHU POINT

The small intestine Shu point is located on the lower back on the pelvis, at the top of the sacrum. From the small of the back, allow your hand to go downward to the edge of the pelvic bone, or the iliac crest. Go three finger-widths (roughly to width of the last segment of your index finger) farther down, and two finger-widths out from the spine, and you will find Bl 27. This is the small intestine Shu point. Feel for any signs of tension or inflammation. Because this is a bony area, you will probably find that the tension is more localized.

As you release these areas, you should occasionally massage down the back and on the back of the legs along the bladder meridian. Spend extra time gently releasing the area behind the knee on point Bl 40, which is very helpful in releasing the back. To find it exactly, bend the knee and put your thumb or finger into the depression behind the knee. When you straighten the knee, you will find that you are actually on a small mound; this is directly behind the joint space. Make sure that you are exactly in the middle of the back of the knee.

Kidney Meridian

If one were to ask a Chinese medical doctor which three organs are the most important in the body, he or she would probably say the liver, spleen, and kidneys.

To both the Western and the Eastern ways of thinking, the kidneys are essential to life, though each maintains this view for slightly different reasons. Because of the kinds of foods we eat, and the pace at which we live our lives, most of us today have weakened kidneys.

By clearing the kidney meridian, working each day on its key points, you can boost the Qi flow to the organs. Thus the kidneys can be strengthened substantially and all the symptoms related to weak kidneys can be reduced or eliminated.

Below is a list of common symptoms associated with disharmony in the kidneys and kidney meridian.

Common Physical Symptoms of Imbalance

Bones achy or weak

Cold extremities (especially the feet)

Darkness under eyes

Drowsiness, lack of energy

Diarrhea

Dizziness on standing (head rush)

Ears ring (tinnitus)

Edema

Hearing loss

Low back pain

Irregular menstruation

Premenstrual syndrome

Reproductive problems

Soles of feet painful or hot

Urinary incontinence

Sexual problems

Hypertension

Hair loss

Common Emotional Symptoms of Imbalance

Fearful, easily frightened

Chronic anxiety

Foolhardiness

THE KIDNEY: FROM WEST AND EAST

The kidneys are paired organs found in the middle back. They are about five inches long and weigh approximately a third of a pound each.

The kidneys are recognized in Western medicine as performing several vital functions. They filter toxins (such as uric acid) from the blood; regulate substances in the blood that we need for health (such as sodium and other electrolytes); convert vitamin D into a usable hormone; and maintain our acid-alkaline balance. Once the waste is accumulated, the kidneys excrete it through the creation of urine, which passes to the bladder via the two ureters. Needless to say, the kidneys are essential to life, though we can survive with only one of them.

In Chinese medicine, the kidneys are responsible for the deep strength and constitutional vitality of the body. They control the Jing, or essential energy, within each cell of the body, and thereby maintain the health, vitality, and function of every organ, system, and sense. This job is so important that the Chinese regard the kidneys as the source of life. Kidney deficiency, or a deficiency of Jing, manifests as low energy, inability to fully mature, premature aging, or senility.

The kidneys are also seen as the root, or source, of the human will. Our capacity to concentrate on a goal, and follow through regardless of obstacles is dependent on the strength of our kidneys.

Together with the bladder, the kidneys govern the balance and movement of fluids in the body. The kidneys also filter waste from the blood. They fulfill the miraculous feat of removing poisonous elements from the blood and then either restoring or eliminating them through the urine. The body's cells are thereby nourished and cleansed by the kidneys.

The kidneys also govern the bones, teeth, and hair on the head (the last things to decay when we die), the reproductive organs, and our inner ear and hearing. Weak kidneys are unable to send sufficient Qi to the inner ear, causing wax buildup, cellular refuse, and atherosclerosis, all of which injure our hearing.

FINDING AND TREATING THE KIDNEY MERIDIAN

The kidney meridian (Ki) starts at the little toe and crosses under the foot to the inner edge of the instep. It circles the ankle bone toward the heel, then rises along the inside of the calf to the inner thigh. At the pubic area, it goes internal for a short distance and reemerges to climb over the abdomen and chest to the collarbone.

When working on the kidney meridian, we are addressing both acute (short-term) obstructions to the flow of Qi and chronic (long-term) blockages that reflect a deep, internal imbalance. Points in an acute condition are more tender and sensitive and will announce themselves—either as pain or heat or as inflammation—almost immediately upon your touch. Points that have been blocked chronically can be more difficult to find, but in any case exist below layers of tension and congestion. (See chapter 4 for a fuller explanation of acute and chronic conditions.)

Remember, as you work gently with either acute or chronic points, you are using yin and yang to disperse areas that are excessive and to build up areas that are deficient.

RELEASING THE KIDNEY MERIDIAN

Begin by tracing the meridian. Then, as described in chapters 3 and 4, you will "release" the meridian by applying moderate pressure on each of the sensitive points until the tension dissipates and the energy flows from the point once again.

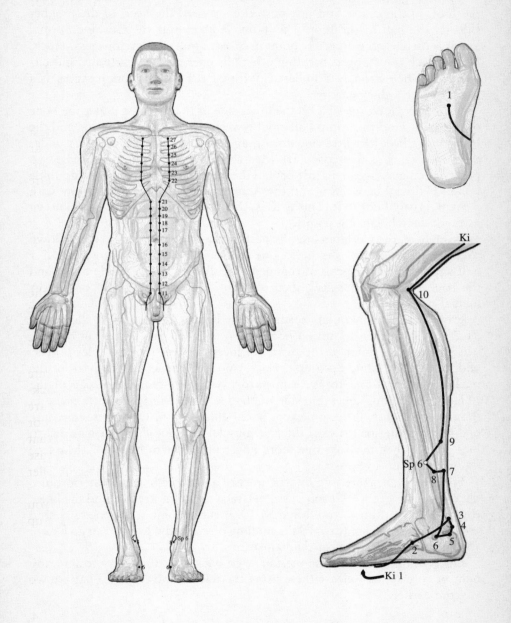

THE KIDNEY MERIDIAN

The first point of the kidney meridian, Ki 1, is located on the bottom of the foot, in the center and just posterior (toward the heel) to the tougher skin on the ball of the foot. This point is known as the Gushing Spring, and it is used as an emergency point in cases of loss of consciousness, shock, heart attack, or stopped breathing. It pulls energy out of storage and circulates it when strongly stimulated. With gentler stimulation, it serves as a tonic for the kidney energy.

From here, look for Ki 2 on the inner side of the foot just under the bone of the arch. Find the bump halfway between the end of the big toe and the back of the heel (the first cuneiform), and go just behind it and just under the bone (which is the navicular). Massage the meridian between these two points; then massage up to just behind the medial malleolus (the inside ankle bone). Halfway between it and the Achilles tendon there is a hollow with a small, gristly knot in it. This is Ki 3, the kidney source point (also known as the kidney balancing point).

From here, the meridian literally performs a loop, dropping directly down to Ki 4 at the top of the heel bone (the calcaneus), then down to Ki 5 halfway between the peak of the medial malleolus (inside ankle bone) and the back corner of the heel, then over to Ki 6 one-half finger below the medial malleolus.

From here, the meridian heads up just behind the medial malleolus to Ki 7 and Ki 8, then to Spleen 6. Spleen 6 is called the Three Yin because it is the meeting point of the three yin meridians of the leg—spleen, liver, and kidney. Let's find Sp 6 first. Place your little finger on the peak of the medial malleolus and measure upward five fingers along the edge of the tibia (the shinbone) on the inside of the leg. You will feel a little niche in the bone, which will be somewhat sore—this is Sp 6. From here, measure one finger posterior (toward the calf muscle) and one finger downward to locate Ki 8, then measure one more finger posterior to find Ki 7. Massage the meridian up to Sp 6.

From Sp 6, measure two fingers upward and three fingers posterior, into the calf muscle, to Ki 9. From here, massage up to the area behind the knee. If you bend your knee, you'll find Ki 10. It is the point in the crease behind the knee as far medial (toward the midline of the body) as you can go before you hit the large tendon of the hamstrings.

Once you have traced the meridian, go back over it and try to find any tight or sore spots. Release these using the release and dispersal pattern we covered earlier.

Key Points on the Kidney Meridian

Ki 1   "Gushing Spring," for infertility, kidney pain, nervous system disorders, calming the spirit. Builds the kidneys and the Jing.

Ki 3   "Great Stream," for any kidney problems; reproductive problems; insomnia. Kidney source point.

Ki 6   "Luminous Spring," along with Bl 60, for releasing the shoulders and neck.

Ki 8   "Junction of Faithfulness," for menstrual disorders; lower back pain and stiffness; building will and confidence.

In addition to clearing the points described above, you can also use the alarm point to disperse excess energy within the meridian, and the Shu point to boost energy to the organ itself.

THE KIDNEY ALARM POINT

The kidney alarm point is the only alarm point located on the back of the body. Find the bottom of the rib cage at the outer edge of the back. Slide medially (toward the middle of the body) from below this rib, which is the eleventh rib, until you reach the tip of the twelfth rib, about two fingers in. This is GB 25, the kidney alarm point. Massage the area relatively gently; you can actually massage from here in to the kidney Shu point (see below) for a more complete kidney release.

THE KIDNEY SHU POINT

The kidney Shu point, Bl 23, is located in the small of the back, between the bottom of the ribs and the top of the hips (the iliac crest). Find the bottom of the ribs on the outside of the back, just in from the sides, and trace a line from there straight across to the spine. You should be on a bone, the spinous process of the second lumbar vertebra. The spinous process is like a tail on the back of the vertebra. Go down to the space between this spinous process and the third lumbar spinous process and move two fingers out from the spine to the kidney Shu point.

Massage this area deeply; notice if one side is fuller than the other and work more on that side, in order to promote proper alignment. As you release this area, you should occasionally massage down the back and on the back of the legs along the bladder meridian. Spend extra time in the area behind the knee on the point Bl 40, which is very helpful in releasing the back. To find it exactly, bend the knee and put your thumb or finger into the depression behind the knee. When you straighten the knee, you will find that you are actually on a small mound; this is directly behind the joint space. Make sure that you are exactly in the middle of the back of the knee.

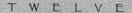

Bladder Meridian

The bladder is one of those organs that we don't think much about until it gives us trouble. Like the rest of the body, the bladder demands adequate life force, or Qi, to function properly. The bladder depends on the kidneys for its health and strength. While we consider bladder infections strictly limited to the organ itself, Chinese medicine sees such disorders as originating in the kidneys, where toxins have not been adequately filtered. Such toxins become the basis for irritations or infections in the lower organ.

By using acupressure to clear the bladder meridian and boost Qi flow to both the kidneys and bladder, you will be giving the bladder exactly what it needs to heal and be restored to good health. Use the techniques and points provided below to strengthen and restore the bladder.

Below is a list of symptoms commonly associated with disharmonies of the bladder and bladder meridian.

Common Physical Symptoms of Imbalance

Back problems

Bladder infection

Incontinence

Hip or sacrum problems

Mania, paranoia

Pain on inside corner of eye

Shoulders rounded

Spasms or pain at back of calf

Feet hurt after standing

Little toe stiff

Common Emotional Symptoms of Imbalance

Jealousy

Long-standing grudges

Excessive suspicion

Fear

Chronic anxiety

THE BLADDER: FROM WEST AND EAST

The bladder is a round sac composed of three layers of muscle. It is located in the lower abdomen, behind the pubic bone.

Western medicine views the bladder's role as fairly straightforward. The bladder stores and secretes urine—it holds about a pint of liquid waste— that originates from the kidneys. As the bladder fills with urine and expands, it sends signals through the spinal cord to the brain, creating the impulse to urinate.

In Chinese medicine, the bladder is part of a system that includes the kidneys and reproductive organs. But more than that, the bladder meridian provides Qi not only to the kidneys but to all the acupressure points on the back—the Shu points—for all the other organs that are on the bladder meridian. It is thereby essential to the entire system. By boosting the Qi to the bladder meridian, you strengthen not only the bladder itself, but every organ in the body.

FINDING AND TREATING THE
BLADDER MERIDIAN

The bladder meridian (Bl) begins at the inside corner of each eye, passes over the forehead and the top of the head, and continues down the back in four lines, two on either side of the spine. The four lines continue over the buttocks and down the legs, where two meet behind each knee. A single line then passes down each leg along the center line of the calf, behind the outer ankle, and ends at the outer tip of the little toe.

When working on the bladder meridian, we are addressing both acute obstructions to the flow of Qi and chronic blockages that reflect a deep, internal imbalance. Points in an acute condition are more tender and sensitive and will announce themselves—either as pain or heat or as inflammation—almost immediately upon your touch. Points that have been blocked chronically can be more difficult to find, but in any case exist below layers of tension and congestion. (See chapter 4 for a fuller explanation of acute and chronic conditions.)

Remember, as you work gently with either acute or chronic points, you are using yin and yang to disperse areas that are excessive and to build up areas that are deficient.

RELEASING THE BLADDER MERIDIAN

Begin by tracing the meridian. Then, as described in chapters 3 and 4 you will "release" the meridian by applying moderate pressure on each of the sensitive points until the tension dissipates and the energy flows from the point once again.

Start by massaging the meridian from the end point, Bl 67, at the outside of the nail on the fifth toe. Massage up the toe between the outside and the top until you are at the lower part of the base knuckle of the fifth toe, pressing Bl 66 where the shaft and knuckle meet. Then go up just over the knuckle and press Bl 65 where the shaft of the fifth metatarsal bone and the knuckle meet.

From here, massage along the outside edge of the fifth metatarsal, moving toward the ankle. A little less than halfway to the ankle, you will reach a bump, which is the proximal end of the fifth metatarsal. Just before this bump is Bl 64, the source point.

To find the next two points, you need to locate Bl 62 first, which is a half finger below the lateral malleolus (outside ankle bone). Bladder 63 is located exactly halfway between Bl 62 and Bl 64 in a small depression. Moving on, Bl 61 is located halfway between the peak of the lateral malleolus and the back corner of the heel. Above that, find Bl 60 behind the lateral malleolus, halfway between it and the Achilles tendon.

From here, massage up the leg just behind the outer edge of the fibula bone, on the outside of the calf muscles. Bladder 59 is located five fingers above Bl 60. Four more fingers up is Bl 58, in a hollow area on the outside of the calf muscles. Bladder 57 is located two fingers diagonally up and in from Bl 58, toward the center of the back of the leg about halfway from the ankle to the knee. Bladder 56 is three fingers up from here, and Bl 55 is four fingers up from Bl 56.

At this point, you should be two fingers below the crease on the back of the knee. (Don't worry if you aren't that close; try measuring backward down the leg to find Bl 55, 56, and 57.) If you bend the knee at a forty-five degree angle and put your thumb up into the center of the hollow created, you will be on Bl 40, a wonderful point for releasing the back which we use repeatedly when working on the Shu points. Outside of Bl 40, just before the lateral tendon of the hamstring muscles, is Bl 39. One finger up from here is Bl 38. We should also note that Ki 10, a kidney point, is just inside of Bl 40, before the medial tendon of the hamstrings.

Once you have traced the meridian, go back over it and find any tight or sore spots. Release these using the release and dispersal pattern we covered earlier, and also release the source point again.

Key Points on the Bladder Meridian

Bl 40   "Entrusting Middle," for leg muscle spasm; knee problems. Helpful point to release the back and shoulders when working with all Shu points.

Bl 60   "Kunlun Mountain," with Ki 6, for strengthening and releasing the back and shoulders. For difficult childbirth.

Bl 62   "Extending Vessel," for nervous system disorders; insomnia; head and eye problems.

Bl 64   "Central Bone," for headache; neck stiffness; back pain. Bladder source point.

In addition to the points described above, you may also use the bladder alarm and Shu points to assist in the healing of the organ. The alarm point can be used to disperse excess energy, and the Shu point can be stimulated to boost energy to the organ.

THE BLADDER ALARM POINT

To find the bladder alarm point, find the middle of the top of the pubic bone and measure three fingers above it. As you can imagine, pressing on this point with any amount of force when the bladder is full can be uncomfortable. Press relatively gently and release and disperse the area with some clockwise rotation.

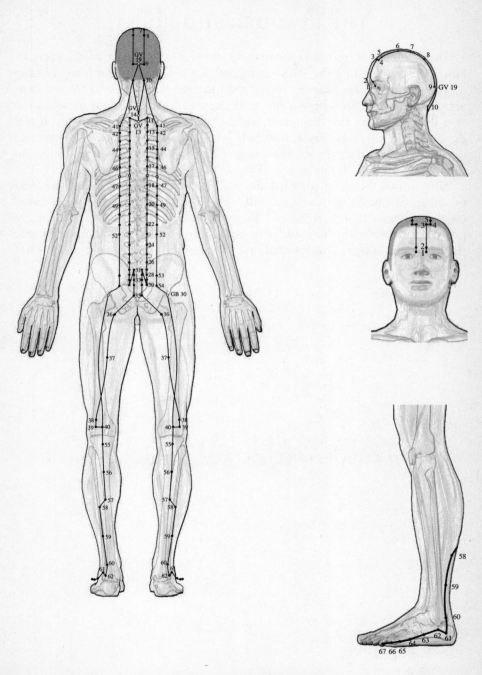

THE BLADDER MERIDIAN

THE BLADDER SHU POINT

The bladder Shu point is located on the second segment of the sacrum. Find it by first finding the PSIS—the posterior superior iliac spine—a bump on the iliac crest. Feel for the top of the hip near the spine and trace downward and inward to where it meets the sacrum, a bony plate between the two ilia that form the iliac crest, at the bottom of the spine. As you feel down, about three fingers below belt level and about a finger below and outside of the top of the sacrum, you will find a relatively large bump on the iliac crest. This bump is the PSIS.

Now move medially (toward the midline of the body) one finger and move down one finger and you will be on the bladder Shu point, located on the sacrum. If it is tight and knotted, you can assume that there are problems either with the bladder or with nerves in the pelvic area. Release the point if it is tight and knotted, and disperse if it is very sore or feels hot to the touch.

Lung Meridian

The lungs grab hold of oxygen from the air and release carbon dioxide, which is the waste from our cellular metabolism. Everyone knows that we need oxygen to survive, but few people realize why we need it: Oxygen is a source of energy.

Many people suffer from respiratory problems today, not the least of which are bronchitis, pneumonia, asthma, emphysema, and lung cancer. All of these are serious illnesses which spring from a single cause: inadequate Qi flow to the lungs and other organs within the body.

You can boost Qi to the lungs by clearing the meridian on a regular basis, stimulating the points I have listed below. By doing so, you will increase the health and vitality of your lungs and your entire body. You'll also breathe a whole lot easier.

Below is a list of disorders that arise when the lungs and lung meridian are in disharmony.

Common Physical Symptoms of Imbalance

Asthma

Bronchitis

Pneumonia

Chest congestion

Coughing

Difficulty breathing

Excessive mucus

Sore throat

Voice loss

Deficient or excessive perspiration

Collapsed or hollow chest

Common Emotional Symptoms of Imbalance

Chronic or long-term grief, sorrow

Compulsive behaviors

Claustrophobia

Restlessness

THE LUNGS: FROM WEST AND EAST

We have two lungs, weighing together about two and a half pounds. They are located under the rib cage, extending from the bottom rib almost to the collarbone.

Western medicine views the lungs as the primary organs of respiration, supplying the body with oxygen and ridding the body of carbon dioxide—essential for energy and life. They are composed of a thick mesh of capillaries whose purpose is to pass oxygen into blood cells.

In Chinese medicine, the lungs are the rulers of Qi; they receive Qi, change it, and disburse it throughout the body. How deeply we breathe shapes the Qi and gives it definition—a nervous, shallow breather will experience the same erratic energy and tend to exhibit a nervous, insecure personality; conversely, a deep, rhythmic breather will have more vitality in his life and expression.

The Chinese believe that the lungs and the heart have a close and important relationship. The lungs, as they take in vital oxygen, give the body energy and make life possible by passing oxygen to the blood that the heart is pumping. At the same time, the heart controls the lungs, balancing the raw energy created by the lungs.

The lungs are also paired, say the Chinese, with the large intestine. Problems affecting one affect the other. When the lungs are irritated by toxins, excess mucus is produced. Toxins not removed by the large intestine enter the bloodstream and find their way into the lungs. Consequently, in Chinese medicine, the lungs are often treated by healing the large intestine.

The emotions associated with the lungs are grief and sorrow, and I would add the quality of acceptance and letting go. When lung energy is in excess, we see excessive acceptance, the "everything's okay with me" syndrome. When the lungs are deficient, we see lack of acceptance, stubbornness, and denial.

FINDING AND TREATING THE LUNG MERIDIAN

The lung meridian (Lu) runs from deep in the body at the lung to surface in the hollow area by the front shoulder. Next it passes over the shoulder and down the front of the arm along the outside of the biceps muscle. It goes down the arm to the wrist just below the base of the thumb, then ends at the thumbnail.

When working on the lung meridian, we are addressing both acute (short-term) obstructions to the flow of Qi and chronic (long-term) blockages that reflect a deep, internal imbalance. Points in an acute condition are more tender and sensitive and will announce themselves—either as pain or heat or as inflammation—almost immediately upon your touch. Points that have been blocked chronically can be more difficult to find, but in any case exist below layers of tension and congestion. (See chapter 4 for a fuller explanation of acute and chronic conditions.)

Remember, as you work gently with either acute or chronic points, you are using yin and yang to disperse areas that are excessive and build up areas that are deficient.

RELEASING THE LUNG MERIDIAN

Begin by tracing the meridian. Then, as described in chapters 3 and 4, you will "release" the meridian by applying moderate pressure on any of the sensitive points until the tension dissipates and the energy flows from the point once again.

Let's start with Lung 11, located on the anterior (away from the index finger) side of the base of the thumbnail. From here, move up to the middle of the bony eminence halfway between the wrist and the first knuckle of the thumb. This is Lu 10. From here, move to Lu 9, which is at the crease of the wrist, at the end of the radius (the bone on the thumb side of the forearm). You will be just lateral (outside) of a tendon.

From here, Lu 8 is located one finger toward the elbow, and Lu 7 is located one more finger farther. To find Lu 6, let's find Lu 5 first. Lung 5

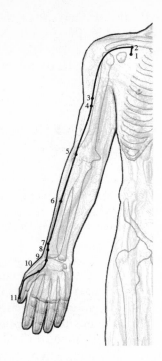

THE LUNG MERIDIAN

is at the inside crease of the elbow on the thumb side. Lung 6 is located five fingers down toward the wrist.

Once you have traced the meridian, go back over it and find any tight or sore spots. Release these using the release and dispersal pattern we covered earlier, and also release the source point again.

Key Points on the Lung Meridian
(See illustration and Point Locator in appendix for locating points.)

Lu 1 "Central Palace," for all lung disorders, chest tightness, upper body heat. Lung alarm point.

Lu 5 "Cubit Marsh," for regulating the lungs, chest tightness, upper body heat.

Lu 7 "Broken Sequence," for colds, nasal blockage, lung congestion, sore throat.

Lu 9 "Great Abyss," lung source point for building and balancing the lungs. For congestion, cough, chest pain, palpitations, irritability, unconsciousness.

In addition to clearing the meridian, you can also stimulate the alarm point to disperse excess energy within the meridian, and the Shu point to boost energy to the organ itself.

THE LUNG ALARM POINT

To find the lung alarm point, put your ring finger just below the clavicle and slide over until you reach the edge of the shoulder joint. From here, measure two fingers (to the index finger) toward the center line, then measure two fingers down from here and you'll will be on Lu 1, the lung alarm point.

THE LUNG SHU POINT

To find the lung Shu point, find the top inside corner of the shoulder blade and trace directly over to the spine. You will be on the spinous process of the second thoracic vertebra. Move down to the space between the second and third thoracic vertebrae and out two fingers to the lung Shu point.

FOURTEEN

Large Intestine Meridian

A *great percentage of the* Western world suffers from problems related to the large intestine, as evidenced by the booming laxative and antidiarrheal industries. Little do we realize that what we really suffer from is a lack of Qi flowing to the large intestine, small intestine, stomach, and spleen. You can remedy that, and in the process clear up your digestive and intestinal disorders, by regularly clearing your large intestine meridian and stimulating the pathway's key points.

Below are an array of symptoms related to disharmonies of the large intestine and large intestine meridian.

Common Physical Symptoms of Imbalance

Constipation

Diarrhea

Headache

Shoulder pain

Nasal congestion

Toothache

Common Emotional Symptoms of Imbalance

Excessive worry

Chronic grief, sadness

Compulsive attention to detail

Stubbornness

THE LARGE INTESTINE: FROM WEST AND EAST

The large intestine is approximately two inches in diameter and six feet long. It has a horseshoe shape and surrounds the many bends of the small intestine. It consists of four parts: the ascending colon, which connects to the small intestine; the transverse colon, which crosses below the diaphragm; the descending colon, which travels down toward the bowel; and the sigmoid colon, which is the pelvic part of the intestine ending with the anus.

The primary function of the large intestine, according to Western medicine, is to receive waste from the small intestine, remove any excess water and nutrients from the feces, and, through peristalsis, move the waste along to the anus, where it is eliminated from the body.

Chinese medicine recognizes that the large intestine performs this function of elimination in its most obvious sense—and it also sees the intestine's function of elimination in a larger, more metaphorical sense. That is, the large intestine's condition reflects the body and mind's capacity to eliminate those experiences, emotions, old beliefs, and patterns we no longer need, so that we can grow and develop as human beings.

The large intestine is also responsible for sending energy downward into the body, and thus grounding us to the earth. As I will describe in depth in chapter 25, "The Five Elements," the organ is paired with the lungs, and together the two are regarded as the Metal Element. Most respiratory and sinus disorders are related to weaknesses in the large intestine function. Similarly, problems with the neck, shoulders, and mouth area are also regarded as linked to imbalances within the large intestine.

FINDING AND TREATING THE LARGE INTESTINE MERIDIAN

The large intestine meridian (LI) starts on the index finger at the outside of the nail (toward the thumb), runs through the crease between the thumb and index finger, and passes up the thumb-side edge of the arm to the edge of the shoulder. Next the meridian crosses the shoulder and neck to the cheek, touches the upper lip, and ends at the nostril.

When working on the large intestine meridian, we are addressing both acute (short-term) obstructions to the flow of Qi and chronic (long-term) blockages that reflect a deep, internal imbalance. Points in an acute condition are more tender and sensitive and will announce themselves—either as pain or heat or as inflammation—almost immediately upon your touch. Points that have been blocked chronically can be more difficult to find, but in any case exist below layers of tension and congestion. (See chapter 4 for a fuller explanation of acute and chronic conditions.)

Remember, as you work gently with either acute or chronic points, you are using yin and yang to disperse areas that are excessive and to build up areas that are deficient.

RELEASING THE LARGE INTESTINE MERIDIAN

Begin by tracing the meridian. Then, as described in chapters 3 and 4, you will "release" the meridian by applying moderate pressure on any of the sensitive points until the tension dissipates and the energy flows from the point once again.

Begin at Large Intestine 1, located on the thumb-side base of the nail of the index finger. From here, move up to the base knuckle, between the top and the thumb side. Large Intestine 2 is located just before the base knuckle; LI 3 is located just after.

Large Intestine 4 is this meridian's source point; it is also considered one of the two most important points in acupuncture or acupressure. It is often used for headaches and intestinal problems, but it is a general tonic for the entire digestive and immune systems. If you squeeze your thumb and first finger together, you'll notice that the webbing swells out the most in a particular spot. If you place your other thumb on that spot, then open your finger and thumb again, you will be on the traditional location for LI 4.

In Integrative Acupressure, we use a slightly different location. Starting with your thumb in the webbing and pointed toward the wrist, move your thumb as far as you can to where the metacarpal bones of the thumb and index finger meet. Press into the side of the second metacarpal, and you'll notice the point. This is the Integrative Acupressure location for LI 4; I find this to be a more effective location when using fingers instead of needles.

From here, slide straight up to the wrist and you'll find a depression

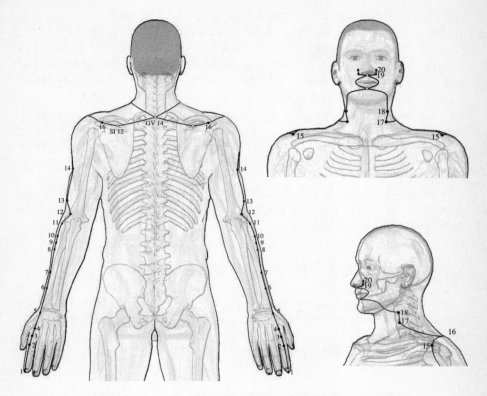

THE LARGE INTESTINE MERIDIAN

between two tendons, which is where LI 5 is located. Five fingers up from LI 5, on the edge of the radius bone, is LI 6. From there, two fingers up, is LI 7. Three fingers above that is LI 8; two fingers above that is LI 9; and two fingers above that is LI 10. To find LI 11, hold your arm as if it were in a sling, then follow across the top of your forearm (the radius) toward the elbow until you are stopped by the joint. Go back one finger and press down into the radius to find LI 11. This is a good point, in combination with LI 4, for treating constipation and for stimulating the immune system.

Once you have traced the meridian, go back over it and find any tight or sore spots. Release these using the release and dispersal pattern we covered earlier, and also release the source point again.

Key Points on the Large Intestine Meridian

LI 4   "Adjoining Valleys," especially when coupled with LI 11, for boosting immune system and digestive organs. For any illness; fever; headaches; voice loss; difficult childbirth; eye disorders; nasal blockage. Large Intestine source point. *No strong stimulation during pregnancy*, because it could stimulate abortion.

LI 10   "Arm Three Miles," for building endurance; regulating digestion.

LI 11   "Crooked Pool," especially when coupled with LI 4 for boosting immune system. For rashes; allergies; acute lower back pain.

In addition to the points described above, you may also stimulate the large intestine alarm point to disperse excess energy and the Shu point to boost energy to the organ.

THE LARGE INTESTINE ALARM POINT

The large intestine alarm point is located three fingers out from the navel, on both sides. Place your index finger in the navel and measure out laterally to the little finger.
Probe and massage these areas gently.

THE LARGE INTESTINE SHU POINT

The large intestine Shu point is located at the bottom of the spine, just above the sacrum. Feel down the outside of the spine until you reach the bottom where it meets the sacrum. You should find two bumps just to the outside of the spine on the iliac crest; this is the PSIS (posterior superior iliac spine). Go just inside this and up one finger to find the large intestine Shu point.

Circulation/ Pericardium Meridian

*The circulation/pericardium mer-*idian, does not directly correspond to an organ but provides Qi to the heart. For this reason it is sometimes described as the "heart's ambassador," the "heart protector," and the "heart governor." All these names illustrate the meridian's role in protecting the heart and nervous system; in Chinese medical practice, it is considered to be an extension of the heart.

Common Physical Symptoms of Imbalance

Stiffness or spasm in arm and elbow

Distended chest and ribs

Red face

Discomfort in chest

Excessive laughter

Hot palms

Sexual dysfunction

Painful or swollen underarm

Tension in upper chest

Blurred vision

Painful, stiff head and neck

Common Emotional Symptoms of Imbalance

Timidity

Anxiety

Nervousness

Insensitivity

Rude behavior

CIRCULATION AND THE PERICARDIUM: FROM WEST AND EAST

In Western physiology, the pericardium is the fibrous sac surrounding the heart. It protects the heart from physical damage and from friction, since the heart is constantly moving. Chinese medicine views the circulation/pericardium meridian in a similar role. As the pericardium physically protects the heart, the meridian absorbs heat and protects the heart from attacks of fever. Most of the points on the meridian reduce heat symptoms associated with heart or blood ailments, and the last three are used for high fevers and sunstroke.

The circulation/pericardium meridian has a more general purpose as well, according to Chinese medicine—namely, to bring joy and happiness, to communicate emotions, and to protect the heart from emotional stress. It does this by calming the mind and balancing the emotions.

FINDING AND TREATING THE CIRCULATION/ PERICARDIUM MERIDIAN

To restore balance and health to the circulatory function, proper Qi flow must be established in the circulation/pericardium meridian (C/P).

The circulation/pericardium meridian starts internally at the surface of the heart and emerges just outside each nipple. It follows around the armpit and down the inside of the arm to the wrist, ending at the thumb-side corner of the middle fingernail.

When working on the circulation/pericardium meridian, we are addressing both acute (short-term) obstructions to the flow of Qi and chronic (long-term) blockages that reflect a deep, internal imbalance. Points in an acute condition are more tender and sensitive and will announce themselves—either as pain or heat or as inflammation—almost immediately upon your touch. Points that have been blocked chronically can be more difficult to find, but in any case exist below layers of tension and congestion. (See chapter 4 for a fuller explanation of acute and chronic conditions.)

Remember, as you work gently with either acute or chronic points, you are using yin and yang to disperse areas that are excessive and to build up areas that are deficient.

RELEASING THE CIRCULATION/PERICARDIUM MERIDIAN

Begin by tracing the meridian. Then, as described in chapters 3 and 4, you will "release" the meridian by applying moderate pressure on each of the sensitive points until the tension dissipates and the energy flows from the point once again. The most important points on the circulation/pericardium meridian are between the fingertips and the elbows.

Start by massaging C/P 9, the endpoint of the circulation/pericardium meridian, which is found at the base of the nail of the middle finger, on the thumb side. Massage upward from here to the base of the middle finger and on to the center of the palm to C/P 8. Massage gently, but firmly. Continue up to the center of the inside—or underside—of the wrist. Probe the area until you find a sensitive depression directly in the center of the wrist line. This is C/P 7, the source point, which balances the whole circulation/pericardium meridian. Return here later if it needs more stimulation.

Continue up the middle of the forearm. Three fingers up from C/P 7 is C/P 6, a useful point for controlling nausea and seasickness. Move one wide finger up from C/P 6 to C/P 5, then three fingers to C/P 4. From here, move up to the inside crease of the elbow, halfway between the two sides, and you are on C/P 3.

Now that you have traced the meridian, go back over it and try to find any tight or particularly sensitive points. Release these using the release and dispersal technique. Finally, return to C/P 7 and stimulate the source point for a minute until you feel that the point has been released and the meridian sufficiently stimulated.

Key Points on the Circulation/Pericardium Meridian
C/P 4   "Crevice Gate," for regulating the heart, calming the spirit. For chest fullness, diaphragm tension, nausea.

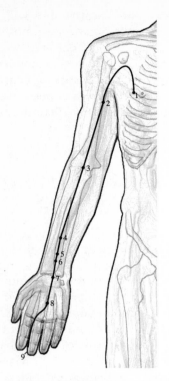

THE CIRCULATION/PERICARDIUM MERIDIAN

C/P 6   "Inner Border Gate," for regulating the heart, calming the spirit. For nausea and seasickness (excellent), balancing the liver and expelling gall stones, facilitating lactation.

C/P 7   "Big Mound," for regulating the heart, calming the spirit. For stomach problems, vomiting, eczema. Circulation/pericardium source point.

In addition to the key points on the meridian, you can also stimulate the alarm point to disperse excessive energy and the Shu point to boost energy to the meridian.

THE CIRCULATION/PERICARDIUM ALARM POINT

The circulation/pericardium alarm point is a four-finger distance below the sternum, directly below the xiphoid process. Massage the area relatively gently, since alarm points are frequently sensitive and often painful. First use the point to determine the degree of imbalance in the meridian: the more acute the pain, the greater the imbalance. Continue to gently stimulate, massaging the point until it is released and the sensitivity or pain is reduced.

THE CIRCULATION/PERICARDIUM SHU POINT

As we discussed in chapter 4, the Shu points are located along the spine and may be used for both diagnosis and treatment. Extremely sensitive Shu points indicate a general deficiency of Qi in the meridian and the related organ. If the circulation/pericardium Shu point is acutely sensitive or painful, disperse the Qi gently using a circular motion. If it is harder and more chronically congested, apply a gentle but deeper pressure to clear the congestion and send Qi into the meridian.

If you are working on yourself, you can stimulate the Shu points by putting two tennis balls into a sock, placing the balls and sock on the floor, and rolling your back on top of them along the spine.

The circulation/pericardium Shu point is located just above the heart Shu point. Find the top of the shoulder blade (scapula) and trace a line from there straight across to the spine. You should be on a bone, the spinous process of the second thoracic vertebra. The spinous process is like a tail on the back of the vertebra; the tip is even with the bottom of the vertebra. Go down to the space between this spinous process and the third thoracic vertebra. The circulation/pericardium Shu point is located two fingers out from here, one wide finger above the heart Shu point.

Check to see if there is any apparent inflammation or tension here. Remember, if the tension is long-term, it will cover the whole area. Feel for a sense of fullness, which prevents you from determining with your fingers any of the details within the layers, such as muscle fibers, bones, or small points.

As you release this area, occasionally massage gently but deeply down the back and on the back of the legs along the bladder meridian. Concentrate your energy and focus in the area behind the knee, on Bl 40, which is very effective at releasing the back.

Triple Warmer Meridian

The Triple Warmer, also known as the "Triple Burner" or "Triple Heater," does not correlate with a specific organ, but rather is seen as a function that controls fluids within the body, most specifically water and the endocrine, or hormonal system. The Triple Warmer derives its name from three centers of activity within the body that, as they function, create heat. These centers and the heat they generate control the body's fluids. The upper warmer is associated with the heart and its fluid, the blood, as well as the lungs and the vaporized air, or mists, within the air; the middle warmer is associated with the liver, spleen, and stomach and the liquefied food matter; and the lower warmer with the kidneys, bladder, and large and small intestines, which also contain even greater amounts of water and liquefied food.

The Triple Warmer is also associated with the endocrine glands, including the pituitary, pineal, thyroid, thymus, pancreas, adrenals, and gonads.

When balanced and functioning well, the Triple Warmer not only regulates these three centers of activity, but coordinates them all so that they function well with each other.

Common Physical Symptoms of Imbalance

Distended or full abdomen

Colds and fevers

Confusion

Deafness and/or pain behind ear

Elbow problems

Eye pain in outer corner

Swollen jaw

Perspiration when sleeping or for no reason

Slow metabolism, overweight

Fast metabolism, hyperactive

Common Emotional Symptoms of Imbalances

None

THE TRIPLE WARMER: FROM WEST AND EAST

There is no clear connection between the Triple Warmer and any Western medical concept, though we can point to the organs associated with each of the three warmers. Chinese medicine describes the three warmers as a pot on a fire. The lower warmer, controlled mainly by the kidneys, is the fire itself. The middle warmer, which controls digestion, is the pot with food in it. The upper warmer, which relates to the breath and vitality, is the steam rising from the pot. If any of the warmers are out of balance individually or with each other, physical disorders arise.

FINDING AND TREATING THE TRIPLE WARMER MERIDIAN

To restore balance and health to the Triple Warmer function, proper Qi flow must be established in the Triple Warmer meridian (TW) by stimulating key points.

The Triple Warmer meridian begins on the outside corner of the nail of the fourth finger and runs up the middle of the outside of the arm to the top of the shoulder. It continues over the shoulder to the collarbone, climbs the back of the neck and circles around the back of the ear, where it continues to the outer corner of the eyebrow.

When working on the Triple Warmer meridian, we are addressing both acute (short-term) obstructions to the flow of Qi and chronic (long-term) blockages that reflect a deep, internal imbalance. Points in an acute condition are more tender and sensitive and will announce themselves—either as pain or heat or as inflammation—almost immediately upon your touch. Points that have been blocked chronically can be more difficult to find, but in any case exist below layers of tension and congestion. (See chapter 4 for a fuller explanation of acute and chronic conditions.)

Remember, as you work gently with either acute or chronic points, you are using yin and yang to disperse areas that are excessive and to build up areas that are deficient.

RELEASING THE TRIPLE WARMER MERIDIAN

Begin by tracing the meridian. Then, as described in chapters 3 and 4, you will "release" the meridian by applying moderate pressure on any of the sensitive points until the tension dissipates and the energy flows from the point once again. The most important points on the Triple Warmer meridian are between the fingertips and the elbows.

Begin massaging the meridian at the outside of the fourth fingernail. From here, massage up to the base knuckle. Just before the base knuckle is TW 2; just onto the back of the hand side of the knuckle is TW 3. From here, massage up to the crease of the wrist; TW 4 is half a finger outside the center of the crease. This is the Triple Warmer source point. Measure three fingers toward the elbow from here to TW 5; this is an important point to stimulate. Triple Warmer 6 is one wide finger up from TW 5; from TW 6 move one finger to the pinky-side to TW 7. Go back to TW 6 and massage a wide finger toward the elbow to TW 8. Four fingers toward the elbow from here is TW 9. Just inside the point of the elbow is TW 10.

Once you have traced the meridian, go back over it and try to find any tight or sore spots. Release these using the release and dispersal pattern covered earlier, and also release the source point, TW 4, again.

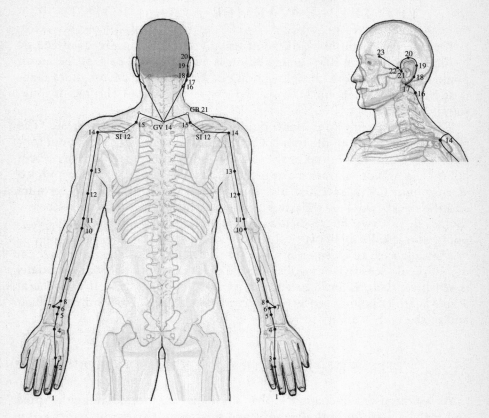

THE TRIPLE WARMER MERIDIAN

Key Points on the Triple Warmer Meridian

TW 4   "Yang's Pool," for colds, fatigue, sore throat, eye redness and swelling. Triple Warmer source point.

TW 5   "Outer Border Gate," for building immunity; dispelling acute illness, headaches, neck stiffness, ear symptoms.

In addition to the key points on the meridian, you can also stimulate the alarm point to disperse excessive energy and the Shu point to boost energy to the meridian.

THE TRIPLE WARMER ALARM POINT

An extremely painful alarm point usually indicates an excess of energy in the meridian, and that the condition is acute. A dull pain at the alarm point indicates a more chronic condition. (See chapter 26 for more diagnostic details.) The point may also be swollen, a sign of chronic or long-standing problems.

There are actually four alarm points related to the Triple Warmer. The first one, starting from the top, is Conception Vessel 17, located about four fingers up from the bottom of the sternum. This is the upper warmer alarm point. The middle warmer alarm point is actually the same as the stomach alarm point: CV 12, located halfway between the bottom of the sternum and the navel. The lower warmer alarm point is located two fingers below the navel. Just two fingers below that is the general Triple Warmer alarm point, about halfway between the navel and the pubic bone.

Massage each of these points and try to determine whether any of them are markedly sensitive or swollen. If one of the three specific warmer points is sensitive, there is an imbalance in its corresponding area. If the general Triple Warmer point is sensitive, there is an imbalance in the entire meridian and in the body's ability to regulate its functions.

THE TRIPLE WARMER SHU POINT

As we discussed in chapter 4, the Shu points are located along the spine and may be used for both diagnosis and treatment. Extremely sensitive Shu points indicate a general deficiency of Qi in a meridian and its related organ. If the Triple Warmer Shu point is acutely sensitive or painful, disperse the Qi gently using a circular motion. If it is harder it is more chronically congested; apply a gentle but deeper pressure to clear the congestion and send Qi into the meridian.

If you are working on yourself, you can stimulate the Triple Warmer Shu point by putting two tennis balls into a sock, placing the balls and sock on the floor, and rolling your back on top of them along the spine.

The Triple Warmer Shu point, Bladder 22, is located outside the first lumbar vertebra. Put your thumbs in the kidney area of the small of the back, about four to five fingers out from the spine, and slide upward until you reach the edge of the ribs. From here, move to a point two fingers out from the spine. This point is associated with the adrenal glands and it often becomes very tight with stress.

Check to see if there is any apparent inflammation or tension here. Remember, if the tension is long-term, it will cover the whole area. Feel for a sense of fullness, which prevents you from determining with your fingers any of the details within the layers, such as muscle fibers, bones, or small points.

As you release this area, occasionally massage gently but deeply down the back and on the back of the legs along the bladder meridian. Concentrate your energy and focus in the area behind the knee, on Bl 40, which is very effective at releasing the back.

To find the point, bend the knee and put your thumb or finger into the depression directly behind the knee. Then straighten the knee; you will find that your finger is on a small mound directly behind the joint. Make sure that you are exactly in the middle of the back of the knee; that's where the point is located.

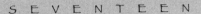

Conception Vessel Meridian

*Though it has no correspond-*ing explanation in Western medicine, the Conception Vessel is seen by the Chinese as the regulator of the peripheral nervous system and, along with the Governing Vessel, controls the other twelve meridians. In addition to providing Qi to all of your peripheral nerves (those outside your spinal column), the Conception Vessel also governs menstruation and the development of the fetus.

Imbalances in the Conception Vessel sometimes manifest as disorders of the peripheral nervous system (shingles, neuropathy), difficulties conceiving and menstruating (such problems may also be related to other meridians, including kidney, liver, Triple Warmer, and circulation/pericardium), and as pain or weakness in the front and middle of the body.

In addition to governing the peripheral nervous system, the Conception Vessel meridian, like the Governing Vessel, does the following:

- Creates balance among the twelve organ meridians, dispersing excess Qi to deficient meridians and areas of the body.

- Unites the organ meridians, allowing Qi flow to adjust when there is a blockage.

- Regulates blood flow in the organ meridians.

Common Physical Symptoms of Imbalance

Asthma

Coughing

Epilepsy

Eczema

Hay fever

Head and neck pain

Laryngitis

Lung problems

Mouth sores and disorders

Pneumonia

Genital disorders

Itching (deficient Qi)

Painful abdominal skin (excess Qi)

FINDING AND TREATING THE CONCEPTION VESSEL MERIDIAN

The Conception Vessel meridian (CV) starts in the pelvic cavity, drops down and emerges in the perineum at a point just between the anus and the genitals. From there, it crosses through the genital area to the top of the pubic bone, runs up the midline of the abdomen, chest, and neck, and ends just below the lower lip.

RELEASING THE CONCEPTION VESSEL MERIDIAN

Begin by tracing the meridian. Then as described in chapters 3 and 4, you will "release" the meridian by applying moderate pressure on each of the sensitive points until the tension dissipates and the energy flows from the point once again.

Begin by massaging along the pathway of the meridian, starting at CV 2, at the pubic bone. The Conception Vessel is most often used as a balancing point, or a kind of anchor, for the practitioner, who typically places one hand on a Conception Vessel point while treating another organ meridian with the other hand. Still, direct massage of the meridian is highly beneficial, starting with CV 2 and working to CV 24, just below the lower lip. Especially emphasize the key points listed below when clearing the meridian, particularly if there appears to be significant congestion along the meridian, and related symptoms of imbalance. Treating the Conception Vessel can be as simple as releasing Lung 7, traditionally referred to as the Conception Vessel meridian's "master point," and Kidney 6, traditionally called the meridian's "coupled point." These points are the equivalent of the source points on the organ meridians.

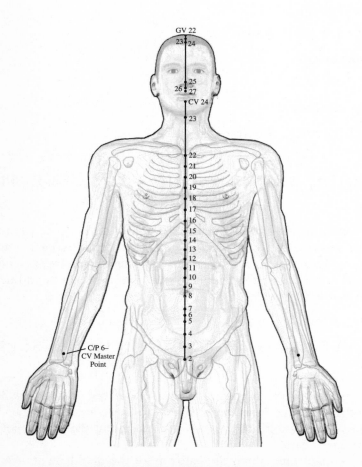

THE CONCEPTION VESSEL MERIDIAN

Key Points on the Conception Vessel Meridian

CV 4, 5, 6 "Hinge at the Source," "Stone Gate," and "Sea of Qi," respectively. For building deep energy, supporting the kidneys, and increasing fertility. These points make up the *dan tian*, or "Cinnabar Field." Cinnabar is the ancient name for mercury, a metal which the ancient Daoist alchemists prized for its near-perfect balance of yin and yang. Cinnabar also refers to a state of balanced consciousness and meditation. The area of the dan tian is considered to be the area that contains our deep-stored energy (Jing).

CV 17 "Central Altar," for balancing the upper warmer, including the lungs and the heart. For all breast disorders.

CV 22 "Heaven's Chimney," for all throat disorders, cough.

Since the Conception Vessel does not correspond to any organ, there are no alarm or Shu points.

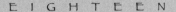

EIGHTEEN

Governing Vessel Meridian

The Governing Vessel does not have a corresponding organ, or even an explanation in Western medical terms. In Chinese medicine, it is the regulator of the nervous system, and, along with the Conception Vessel, it controls the other twelve meridians. It is considered an "extra" meridian by the Chinese.

Imbalances in the Governing Vessel meridian manifest as disorders of the central nervous system, including the brain and spinal cord, as well as the spinal vertebrae.

In addition to governing the nervous system, the Governing Vessel meridian, like the Conception Vessel meridian does the following:

- Creates balance among the various organ meridians, acting as a pressure relief valve, or the floodplain of a river, allowing excess energy to pass through the Governing Vessel, which in turn passes that excess on to other meridians that may currently be deficient of Qi.

- Serves as an adjunct meridian enabling Qi to flow to a particular organ when that organ's meridian is severely blocked.

- Regulates blood flow in the twelve organs.

Common Physical Symptoms of Imbalance

Rounded shoulders, heavy head (deficient Qi)

Headaches and pain in eyes (excess Qi)

Stiffness in spine (excess Qi)

Back pain or tension

Dizziness

Eye problems (including conjunctivitis)

Cold extremities

Fevers

Hemorrhoids

Insomnia

Neck pain

Nervousness or overstimulation

Spinal problems

Common Emotional Symptoms of Imbalance

None

FINDING AND TREATING THE GOVERNING VESSEL MERIDIAN

The Governing Vessel meridian (GV) begins in the pelvic cavity then drops down and emerges below the genital area. It then passes to the tip of the coccyx (tailbone). From here, it moves upward across the sacrum and along the spine, up over the head to the upper lip. Here, it goes under the lip to the upper gum.

RELEASING THE GOVERNING VESSEL MERIDIAN

Begin by tracing the meridian. Then, as described in chapters 3 and 4, you will "release" the meridian by applying moderate pressure on any of the sensitive points until the tension dissipates and the energy flows from the point once again.

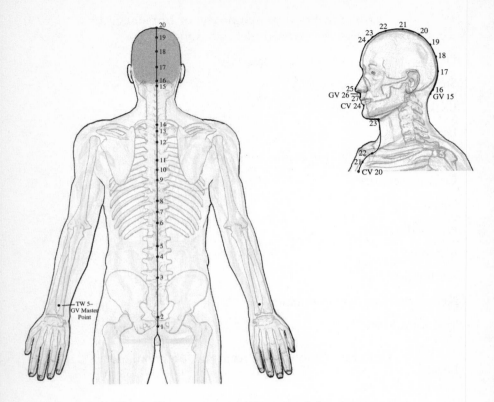

THE GOVERNING VESSEL MERIDIAN

Begin by massaging along the pathway of the meridian, starting at GV 1, at the tip of the tailbone. Although this meridian is most often used as a balancing point for one hand while the other is treating another meridian, direct massage from GV 1 along the key points listed below is useful if there appears to be significant congestion along the meridian and related symptoms of imbalance. Treating the Governing Vessel can be as simple as releasing Small Intestine 3, known as the "master point" for the Governing Vessel meridian, and Bladder 62, known as the meridian's "coupled point."

Key Points on the Governing Vessel Meridian

GV 1   "Lasting Strength," for building the spinal column and central nervous system. For all rectal problems, hemorrhoids, lower back and sacral pain.

GV 14, 15, 16   "Big Vertebra," "Gate of Muteness," and "Wind's Palace," respectively. This whole area is a common entry point for "wind" conditions (discussed in chapter 26), such as cold, damp, or hot drafts that "invade" the body and cause any number of conditions, including stiff neck and shoulders, lung congestion and cough, headaches, fever, and back pain. If the area has been "invaded," it will feel stiff and full, with tension that seems to dissipate but then is back again in a few minutes. Deep, brisk, Qi-moving massage of this whole area, along with hot compresses, can be very helpful for these conditions, especially when treated early.

GV 20   "Hundred Meeting," for clearing the brain, improving memory, any central nervous system disorders, premature graying of hair, ringing in ears. For lower warmer disorders, such as infertility, impotence, urinary incontinence.

GV 26   "Middle of Man," for shock of any sort, loss of consciousness, weeping depression, nasal disorders, chest congestion.

Because there are no specific organs that correlate to the Governing Vessel, and because the meridian is considered an "extra" meridian—an adjunct to the meridian system—there are no alarm or Shu points associated with the Governing Vessel.

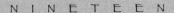

Structure

A thirty-eight-year-old man came to me several years ago with a severe lower back injury that caused radiating pain throughout the lumbar and sacral areas of the back and down the right leg. The lower lumbar area was in such acute pain that my client could not stand up straight and essentially hobbled through the door when he entered. The focal point of the problem was lumbar 5 and sacral 1. The sacroiliac joint in the pelvis had been severely turned so that the right hip was slightly higher than the left. This misalignment also caused his left leg to be longer than his right. The upper back—the cervical and thoracic vertebrae—was loaded with tension, and the lower lumbar had bowed outward, away from the body.

You will recall from my previous discussions of structural alignment issues that when muscles go into spasm, they pull on the spine, causing a zigzag or S-shaped pattern. Either the upper or the lower part of the S-shaped curve is a compensatory response to a severe spasm in the other part of the back, where the problem is most acute. In this client's case, the real problem was in the lumbar area, but there was also a great deal of tension in the upper back. This upper back tension kept the lower back from having the freedom of movement to adjust or correct itself. Naturally, my temptation was to go to the acute area first—in this case, the lumbar area—but that would have been a mistake. The tension, and its accompanying rigidity in the upper back was too great. The moment my client was off the table his lumbar region would return to its earlier deformed shape.

Therefore, I began to work first by releasing the tension in the muscles of the upper back, especially in the right and left sides of the cervical area. I then moved down, releasing the muscles in the thoracic region. I also increased the flow of Qi down the back and the back of the legs, by way of the bladder meridian.

All of this loosened the upper back and took some tension off the lower lumbar region, allowing me to begin working very gently on the most acute tension and pain, in the lumbar vertebrae. I then began to disperse the acute inflammation in the lumbar 5–sacral 1 and sacroiliac joint areas, using our release and dispersal pattern. I did this very gently, because the area was in acute pain.

Once I had cleared enough of the inflammation, I could work more deeply. I released the muscles and points on both sides of the lumbar and sacrum in order to balance the compensatory zigzag pattern of the muscles and structure.

After this first treatment, I was able to work with the lumbar 5–sacral 1 area more deeply and began to clear some of the pressure caused by long-term inflammation and adhesions. Although I was very careful to disperse any areas I released thoroughly, I realized that the client was going to be in treatment for a while to completely clear his system. Within the first few sessions, the client was able to walk upright, although he still had to be very careful. As the acute inflammation cleared, I was able to work more deeply to repair the area and increase balanced mobility.

It took about two months of twice-weekly meetings before he was healthy again. The problem he had was many years old. A recent accident had only triggered the muscles to go into spasm and bring about the acute problem. When those muscles had healed and the Qi was restored in his back, the spine was in a far healthier alignment than it had been before the accident, because the chronic muscle spasms, which he had suffered for many years, had been relieved.

This client's back was worked on regularly for more than a year after his accident and he continues to receive regular acupressure treatments in order to maintain the health of his back. Happily, he has never had an acute injury since, and his back remains healthier today than at any time in his adult life.

When working with any kind of structural issue, such as a back injury or spinal misalignment, there are several principles to keep in mind. In this chapter, I am going to lead you through those principles so that you have an orderly and balanced approach to working with any structural issue.

Eleven principles are essential to the Integrative Acupressure approach to structural work. Many of these principles are the same as we used earlier in the book in relation to energetic work—the clearing of meridians and the boosting of Qi—but we apply them differently when we are working with structure.

1. STRUCTURAL ENERGETICS

When working with structure, keep in mind that the distinction between structure and energetics is a convention to help us understand how the body works; in reality, anytime you are working with structure, you are working with energetics. You can increase structural release by moving energy through the related meridians, and you can increase energy movement in the meridians by structural work. In fact, you will get the best release if you work with both.

For example, imagine you are working on a client's back. You find an area of congestion in the mid back, in the area of the liver Shu point. You could approach it as a structural problem and try to loosen the muscles but what you will probably find is that the area will only release a certain amount—to release more, you have to use excessive pressure to break through the tension. You could also approach it from the energetic perspective and release the points along the bladder meridian to move the congested Qi. This would be productive but slow to take effect.

The best solution is to incorporate both techniques. Release the meridian locally through acupressure, then go to the site of congestion and release the muscular tension. You can facilitate the release even further by mobilizing the area—move the ribs from the side while you work on the tension. By using these two approaches together, you will be able to work easily and quickly, with less pressure. This is important both for the client's comfort and to prevent injury to you.

2. GIVING THE BODY A UNIFORM TONE

A crucial principle of Integrative Acupressure is that it is better to release all areas of the body 65 percent than to release one area 100 percent. There is no difference between everything being uniformly loose or uniformly tight—the body will find its appropriate muscle tone if it is not hindered by structural imbalances and compensations.

You have probably heard of babies who survive unharmed after falls that would have killed most people. Similarly, drunks often survive car accidents far better than if they were sober. The reason is simple: babies and drunks are both loose evenly. They don't have big differences between their tightest and loosest muscles.

The method used in Integrative Acupressure is to release from the tightest muscles to the loosest muscles, one level at a time. Some forms of massage focus only on relaxing the muscles and thereby fail to change the underlying pattern of tension. Integrative Acupressure retrains the body and mind to maintain structural balance.

3. INITIATING GENERAL RELEASE

One common tendency of beginners is to stay in one place for a long time. A novice practitioner may think, "I've found something, and if I move, I'll never find it again." The appropriate pace can only be learned through time and experience. You need to have faith that, if it's important, you'll find it again. Remember that this is not an inert body you are working on. You are developing a communication with your client's body, and it's going to work with you to find all the important spots.

A fundamental assumption of Integrative Acupressure is that the body continues working on an area even when we are not. Remember that you are *initiating* release; you don't need to make an area perfect while you are working on it. In fact, the areas we work on will usually continue to release for two or three days afterwards and often there is more release a week later. So you must learn when you have created enough release to initiate the process. Often, it is much better to spend a few minutes with an area and come back to it later—giving the area time to release and process the change. This will also allow you to identify the tightest areas.

4. NEUROLOGICAL FEEDBACK

Neurological feedback is a useful tool in repatterning the nervous system. Here's an example of using feedback with structural conditions:

Your client has a very tight knot in his lower back, so first you do a quick release of the bladder meridian, which runs down the back, along with Bl 40 behind the knee. Next, you begin to release the point of tension with a sliding motion of the thumb or fingers. If you are using your thumb, it should remain in contact with the same spot on the back, which means that as it slides, the thumb will move in an arc so that the point of contact on your thumb changes, rather than the whole thumb moving to a different point on the back. You might start at the tip of the thumb and slide back to the first knuckle. At the same time, judge how well the area is releasing. If it doesn't release at all, you don't slide your thumb. If it releases slowly, you slide slowly. This gives the person's nervous system (or your own, if you are working on yourself) an exaggerated feedback of how well they are releasing, and supports them to release rather than you forcing them.

Neurological feedback serves three purposes: One, it saves your fingers. Because you are constantly changing the angle of pressure, you don't overstimulate any particular muscle or overirritate any joint. Secondly, you are helping your client to release more easily and eventually to release on his own. Third, it sets up a two-way communication between you and your client's body, enabling you to get information about how "asleep" an area is, and therefore how much you need to work to increase awareness in the area.

5. RECOGNIZING FULLNESS AND EMPTINESS

In structural work, fullness almost always means tight or congested muscles and fascia or tissue adhesions. Generally, you want to work only on the full areas in order to move the congested Qi onward. Otherwise, the balance of the body's structure is thrown off, causing the body to compensate with imbalanced muscle tone.

Remember that fullness means there is less detail, not more. A bone sticking up doesn't mean that an area is full. Imagine you have a bathtub with some large rocks on the bottom, and a large plastic sheet covers the tub. If you were to feel down through the sheet, it would be very easy to grasp the rocks. This is comparable to an empty condition. However, if the bathtub is full, it would be much harder to push through the water to feel the rocks. This is fullness.

Fullness is congested energy, caused by either external or internal forces. External forces include injuries, stressors, or toxins. Internal forces include emotions, organ imbalances, and external conditions that have become chronic and moved deep within the body.

6. CHRONIC AND ACUTE CONDITIONS

The concepts of acute and chronic illness are very straightforward, though frequently misunderstood. The terms chronic and acute simply refer to the duration of a condition. *Chronic* comes from the Greek word *khron-*

ikos and the Latin word *chronicus*, having to do with time, so chronic illnesses are simply long-term conditions (like allergies or tuberculosis). *Acute* comes from the Greek word *akis* and the Latin word *acus,* meaning "needle" (from which we get acupuncture and acupressure); here, it refers to conditions that are short-term and often intense (such as a cold or flu). Of course, the nature of a long-term condition means that chronic conditions will often be debilitating or even life-threatening, but it is also very possible to die from an acute condition. In other words, the terms *chronic* and *acute* say nothing about the severity of a condition, only its duration.

When practicing structural work, we distinguish between chronic and acute conditions by their activity level. An acute structural imbalance will appear as a hot, sharply painful, and possibly red area—meaning that the body has brought extra energy and resources to deal with the problem. If the acute condition isn't resolved, the body will eventually stop trying and will direct energy elsewhere. Then, the problem has become chronic and is marked by less activity than in the surrounding areas. To treat chronic and acute conditions, we use release and dispersal.

7. RELEASE AND DISPERSAL

I hope the concepts of release and dispersal are starting to seem like old friends by now—we have been talking about them since early in the book. The important thing to remember, in treating structure, is to alternate between release and dispersal. The more you release a chronic area, usually the more "acute" it will become, as the body once again tries to send healing energy. The problem area will become congested with Qi that needs to move, so you will need to disperse it. Conversely, the more you disperse an acute area, the more it will congeal into a chronic knot, so you will need to do some release. In general, the more acute the area, the less you will release and the more gentle your release will be. Likewise, the more chronic an area is, the more "releasive" you will need to be.

For example, picture two different conditions—a muscle spasm and a bad bruise—and how you would treat them. With the muscle spasm, you are working to break up tension and get in deeper, waking the area up. It is more likely to be a chronic condition. With a bruise you would probably want to start around the edge of the irritation and gently encourage the flow of blood and Qi out of the area, calming and spreading the energy.

You will repeat this "release and disperse" cycle over and over in a treatment. The art in this process is knowing when to do each. How will you know? Your fingers will show you if you will let them. They will unerringly disperse when the area is soft, warm, and squishy and release when there is any chronic, hard congestion—as long as your conscious mind doesn't get in the way by saying, "I know what to do. I know what this area needs."

At this point in Integrative Acupressure training, students often ask, "If release and dispersal are more intuitive than intellectual, then how do they *feel* different from each other?" Release feels more like you are moving inward, focusing energy and bringing awareness to the area. Dispersal is more calming, spreading—distributing energy outward. Use your conscious mind to form each of these images as you are treating, and the fingers will find the proper pressure and direction.

8. THE THREE LAYERS

The way that you work with an area, whether to release or to disperse, will also depend on which "layer" is involved. Earlier, we discussed three layers of tension—flat surface tension, second-layer bands or ropes, and third-layer knots or points. Understanding this concept is essential to working with structure.

THE FIRST LAYER

The first layer of tension consists of *planes* on the surface of the body— like armor protecting an area. This is the most important tension to release, because it is the most severe. The first layer prevents the release of the other two layers underneath it. It most reflects external stresses, injuries, and acute illnesses. Fortunately, this is also the layer on which massage generally works best.

Many people don't notice first-layer tension and instead tend to focus on the knots and bands of second- and third-layer tension. The problem with this approach is that almost certainly, the original site of inflammation is in the first layer and the other layers are merely compensating for it. Compensating muscles are usually the most painful areas and therefore cry out for attention, whereas the original problem may be completely dormant. So beware the temptation to work on the painful, knotted area—you may thus run the risk of overlooking the "hidden" original problem. You must focus your treatment on the original problem area, rather than on the area that the nervous system tightened in response.

Novice bodyworkers also often mistake first-layer tension for no tension—because they don't feel any distinct tension—but this is in fact one of the distinguishing characteristics of the first layer: lack of detail. Does this sound familiar? Lack of detail is one of the characteristics of "fullness."

Fullness is stagnant Qi, and *the three layers of tension are different variations of fullness*—specifically they are three different *depths* of fullness.

The Second Layer

The second layer is found deeper in the muscles and ligaments, which shows in its characteristic bands or "lines" of tension. This layer reflects nervous system stress and is created by a combination of external stressors and internal imbalances. Most structural or deep tissue work concentrates here, since this layer *feels* most like what we think of as tension. But if you work on the second-layer tension exclusively, the first-layer tension will compensate and negate the work you have done.

The Third Layer

The third layer consists of acupressure points and the tension and adhesions directly around them. This is the core of the tension, reflecting imbalances at a deep energy/organ level. Third-layer tension acts like seed crystals for the growth of first- and second-layer tension. This deep layer often goes untreated and is therefore frequently the slowest to heal. Of course, the third layer is where acupuncture and acupressure treatments concentrate.

General Approach

Integrative Acupressure works from the first (surface) layer down to the third (deep) layer tension. This order is essential for structural work. The only time to deviate is when you need to work with deeper imbalances directly, without having to release the structural layers first—for example, in treating an urgent functional problem (organ dysfunction, headache, exhaustion, etc.).

As mentioned above, the three layers represent different depths of fullness. Since fullness is a form of congestion (acute or chronic), we can say that the three layers show where the body has been imbalanced—near the surface (protective, nourishing, activating) or deep within (affecting organ, nervous system, and deep-stored energy). Of course, the layers also tell us the relative severity and longevity of the condition because the stronger and longer-lasting a condition is, the more it will affect all three layers. And the more it affects all three layers, the more *primary* it is, meaning it is one of the original problems the body has been trying to balance through the use of compensation.

9. COMPENSATION

Compensation is the nervous system's attempt to adapt to new surroundings, optimize support, and minimize discomfort. Some examples of compensation include walking in high heels, or on a tilted surface, or with an injured leg. Imagine someone struggling to do a lot of chin-ups. At first, the movement is straight and smooth. Then, as the primary muscles wear down, the nervous system compensates by looking for other muscles to do the job, and the person begins to twist and wriggle. Or picture yourself climbing stairs. Your nervous system quickly sets up a pattern of movement based on the height of each stair and plays it back like a tape. If one of the steps is higher than the others, you will probably trip on it.

Within the body, the nervous system is constantly compensating for imbalances. If the muscles are tense and tight in one area (exhibiting fullness), the nervous system will compensate by creating fullness in another area to make balance. We cannot change the underlying pattern of structural imbalance without addressing these compensations.

One of the miracles of the human body is its ability to compensate for injuries and defects. Whenever the body cannot do an activity easily or without pain, the nervous system starts looking for appropriate compensations, ways of moving the body that don't rely as much on the compromised areas. Unfortunately, the *pattern* that the body uses to compensate tends to become a habit. For example, if you had a stone in your shoe, you would walk in a way that favors the painful part of your foot. If for some strange reason you didn't remove the stone for several weeks or months, this pattern of compensation would become relatively permanent. Just removing the stone would not solve the problem; you would need to unlearn the habit, or *repattern,* the nervous system's relationship to the body.

10. REPATTERNING

Repatterning is the process of guiding the nervous system to a revised and more appropriate pattern of support and movement. We can change the way the nervous system and the body interact—by the selective, complementary release of related areas of the body. The end result is a brain that knows how the body works and where the body is in space. This creates much less stress on the body and the brain. For example, how many people walk around with their head tilted to one side? If you get someone on your massage table whose brain thinks her head is straight when it isn't, you have a patient with a great deal of stress on all the joints and muscles of the neck. She also has a changed relationship with all the bones of her skull, and the bite of her teeth. If you tilt your head to one side, your teeth will meet unevenly—try it! Anyone who is familiar with TMJ (temporo-mandibular joint dysfunction) knows how big a problem this can be. Imagine, if we could somehow reset the nervous system so it actually knew where the head was in space, how much less stress there would be.

I had a client once, many years ago—before I had developed my method of repatterning—who was hit by a car as he was walking across a parking lot. After his injuries had healed, his sacroiliac joint remained very painful. By the time he got to me, he had been treated by an orthopedist, an osteopath, and two chiropractors. The story with the last chiropractor told the tale—after an adjustment, he would feel good until getting into his car, or sometimes just getting off the table, then he would feel the joint go out again. The second time I saw him, he was very encouraged—the muscular work I had done had succeeded in maintaining the joint for a whole day. I was discouraged, however, and not just because I was young and inexperienced. I had done my best work with him the week before—if I couldn't do better than one day's relief the first time, I was afraid I wouldn't be able to permanently improve things.

Halfway through the second session—after I had finished most of the structural and muscular work I knew how to do at the time—my client had to get up to relieve himself. When he returned, I was devastated to find that the sacroiliac joint had already begun to move out of place, perhaps 30 percent out compared to when he came in. I reapplied the same techniques I had used before, balancing muscle tone and releasing and dispersing inflammation, and it returned to balance. I said nothing to the client, but I was very discouraged.

The following week when he returned, he was jubilant. It had stayed almost perfect all week! Sure enough, when I checked the joint it was only out a small amount. I realized that I had inadvertently done something right by giving the nervous system a second chance to adapt to the structural changes. This was the beginning of my work with the nervous system and compensatory patterns.

The body has an innate sense of natural and efficient movement. It tends to find the most natural way of moving, but, if it has had very strong or very long-term problems, eventually it will become stuck in a pattern. Pain is perhaps the strongest influence in creating one of these "stuck" patterns; the more pain the person has experienced, especially if it is long-term pain, the more likely that the compensation won't go away when the condition improves. And, in fact, often the compensatory pattern will resist balancing the structure, perpetuating the condition instead, as it did with my client.

In order to reverse this nervous system pattern of movement—to *repattern it*—we mildly "irritate" the muscles that have become overdeveloped and balance the structures that have become misaligned. We don't have to irritate the muscles badly; our normal pattern of release and dispersal will work just fine. We then allow the nervous system a chance to experience movement in this "new" body, then work on the person a bit more to undo the damage to our work.

Over the following days, as our client uses her body, the balanced structure makes it easier to move with more ease and in a way that feels more natural. At the same time, the excessively strong muscles keep sending a message to the brain saying "Gosh, I'm a little sore and tired, I'd rather you didn't use me today." (This soreness is slight enough and spread out enough that most people don't even notice it.) So the nervous system goes to the weaker muscles and has them do more of the work, strengthening them and reinforcing a new pattern of movement. Perhaps you will only be able to shift the pattern somewhat closer to the optimal way of moving in one session, but over time the compensation will continue to dissolve.

I call this treatment *reverse compensation,* the concept of releasing and intentionally weakening an overly strong set of muscles, so that the nervous system and the body develop a more appropriate pattern of compensation. Once the body has been given a more comfortable way of moving, it will use it in lieu of an inferior pattern; however, it must experience moving in this new way a while before it will create and reinforce the new pattern. Consequently, we find that any structural changes we make will tend to backslide as the person begins to move around. It's as though the new pattern and the old pattern are in conflict. Unless we reinforce the new pattern, the old pattern will dilute it and we will end up with only a partial change.

11. REINFORCING THE NEW PATTERN

The final principle combines all of the above in order to make the changes long-lasting. Pattern reinforcement simply involves reinforcement of the pattern by the practitioner—releasing the affected areas again. A simple but effective way to reinforce the new pattern is to have your client get up and walk around for a minute in the middle of a session. The client may initially appear uneven or unsteady on his feet, but after a bit that will go away. If he walks for much longer than a minute, he will usually begin to revert toward the old pattern. Pain or discomfort may begin to return. In any case, have him lie down again. You will find that some of the original imbalance and muscular tension has returned. You can actually tell how severe the condition is by how much of the original condition returns. However, you will also find that it releases much more quickly than the first time, and that the repatterning will be better intact when they get up again. In fact, this one additional repatterning will often mean the difference between maintaining an imbalanced condition and correcting it. Usually, only one repatterning is sufficient but sometimes multiple treatments may be required.

An added complication is that everyone has a practically limitless number of movement patterns, some which are used daily, others that may not be used in over forty years. Each time you sit down, bend over, run, etc., you are utilizing one of these patterns. If we change the structural support of the body, the nervous system will have to change all of these movement patterns, one by one as they are used.

Years ago, I was working with a fellow who had a number of complaints, including lower back pain. After working with him for a few weeks, the back pain seemed to be under control, so I was spending much less time on his back in the sessions. One day, he came in complaining that his back was hurting again. When asked how and where, he replied, "It just feels off, like it used to feel before you worked on it." I asked him the obligatory questions to see if he had somehow strained it; an athletic middle-aged man, he assured me that he had, in fact, had a very relaxed weekend. Then I asked, "Did you do anything which you haven't done in a while?" He brightened and said, yes, he had gone out with an old friend and run football patterns they had used back in college; the back had become problematic by that evening. This had effectively reinforced his old way of holding himself. Fortunately, with a little work and a little "pattern reinforcement," it was as good as new.

HOW PATTERNS ARE BORN

It's important to have a model of how the brain creates and utilizes movement patterns. If you have had the dubious honor of learning to drive a standard shift car, you probably had trouble imagining how anyone could pull out the clutch so smoothly that the car didn't jerk, much less press the accelerator with such precise timing that the car didn't stall and actually moved forward. After practicing for a while, however, the motion becomes so automatic that you don't have to think about it.

When we first learn something new, it is "figured out" in the cerebral cortex, our thinking brain. The cerebral cortex figures out these tasks one at a time. Once it figures out the first part (pulling out the clutch slowly enough that the car doesn't jerk), it passes this over to the cerebellum, which remembers it as a *synergistic pattern* of nerve impulses going out and kinesthetic information from the senses returning.

Synergy occurs when separate elements work together to create something new which is more than each of the parts. The flight of a bird is a synergistic coordination of different movements—without any one part, flight would not occur. The cerebellum sees these movements as a whole, a "package," not as separate parts. Kinesthetic refers to information we get from the efferent nerves, nerves which register our location in space. Without the kinesthetic feedback you get from the efferent nerves, you would stumble a lot, bump into things, and poke yourself in the eye. For its part, the cerebellum is simply "remembering" what is sent out of the brain and what comes back. As you begin to move in a certain way, or anticipate moving in a certain way, the nervous system pulls out the appropriate movement pattern from its archives. The cerebellum plays this back like a tape recorder until and unless the sensory or kinesthetic information coming back is significantly different from what it should be according to the "tape recorder." If the pattern it remembers doesn't match the information coming back in, the nervous system enters "repatterning mode" and modifies the pattern to fit better. You are constantly doing this—modifying your programming for new experiences throughout a lifetime.

HOW PATTERNS GET DILUTED

Although the body is constantly repatterning, it doesn't easily forget the old ones. Let's say that you just had a bodywork treatment and had your hips balanced—your legs, which were different lengths, are now even. You get into your car and put your feet on the pedals. Immediately, your cerebellum starts playing back the "get in the car, push in the clutch, turn the key, and press the accelerator" pattern, but the clutch is a little farther away than it's supposed to be and the gas pedal is, conversely, a little closer. While the brain is modifying its pattern to accommodate the change, the body is also doing some modifying—it's trying to shift back to the old imbalance to accommodate the old pattern. This is what happened to our suffering ex-football player—like putting on twenty-year-old shoes, he put on an old pattern and it didn't fit.

Reinforcing new patterns may be accomplished in several ways. One is, as I described, having the client walk around. Walking is one of the most common movement patterns, and is effective because it is repetitive. Another is directly repatterning the movements that created the problem. Once a client is relatively balanced, I will have them perform the original repetitive movement that created the problem—while I work to release and repattern the problem areas. For example, with carpal tunnel (wrist) clients, I might have them type or play the piano while I release their neck and shoulders, which is usually where the problem is coming from. As the old pattern reinstates, you can feel muscles tightening and the posture changing. I release each muscle as it tightens, effectively saying to the nervous system, "not that way, try another way." If I can't release it enough while they are in motion, I have them stop for a moment while I release the area.

THE WINDOWS OF VULNERABILITY

There are two "windows of vulnerability" during the process of repatterning. One "window" is the period of time just after the treatment. In the hours and days after a treatment, you want the client to avoid strenuous work. Otherwise, the client's nervous system may override the stronger muscles' request to rest; and this will reinstate the old pattern. Another possibility is that the weaker muscles, which aren't used to working so hard, will be overtaxed and possibly strained or injured.

Another "window of vulnerability" happens when you are seeing the client less frequently. Over time, the new movement patterns will become diluted until the person starts having structural problems again. For this reason, it is best to "wean" the client for as long as six months to a year. Typically, when you feel that the client is ready, have him skip a week. If all goes well, then go to every other week for a few sessions. Once the client seems fine with every other week, go to once a month for one or two times. Finally, let the client know that he should return if at any point he feels *anything* to indicate he is off balance, and even if he has no problems, he should return in about six months. It is very important to stress to the client that the sooner he comes back in after a problem, the quicker you will be able to remedy it. If he waits, a problem that might have taken one session to fix will take two or three.

A FINAL NOTE

Keep in mind that with Integrative Acupressure, you don't have to come up with a diagnosis before you put your hands on someone—in fact, the information you receive from your hands is usually the most important part of your understanding. You will do much better work from a place of curiosity and exploration, rather than deciding in advance how the body needs to be healed.

TWENTY

Whole Body Structure Release

WORKING WITH THE TORSO: AN OVERVIEW

When we work with the back and pelvis, we want to start with a broad scope and gradually become more detailed, corresponding to the three layers. At the same time, however, we want to continually step back and see the big picture, like an artist, working close to canvas but needing to keep the whole view in mind. We must address it as a whole rather than seeing the different problems separately.

The back is an interdependent system, where everything balances everything else. If something goes amiss, we can't treat it as an isolated problem. Like a fire which starts in one place and then spreads, any imbalance in the back will have to be balanced by the rest of the back, creating compensations. We need to treat all of these compensations as equally important.

We can do this by addressing the Shu points on the sides that the spine is pulling toward. This means that we must work selectively, and we must be able to tell which sides have the shorter muscles and which have the longer. Fortunately, it is very easy to tell once you have a little bit of experience. We want to feel for fullness and emptiness.

CHALLENGES TO ALIGNMENT

One of the biggest problems with maintaining alignment is the fact that the shorter a muscle is, the stronger it is and the more likely it is to go into spasm (fullness); the longer a muscle is, the weaker it is and the less likely it is to go into spasm (emptiness). Within the back, this means that if a vertebra gets displaced laterally, the muscles on one side will get shorter and stronger and the muscles on the other side will get longer and weaker. Within a certain range, it's quite possible for the nervous system to realign this vertebra simply by tightening the muscles on the opposite side; however, if the vertebra gets too far out of line the opposing muscles will be longer and weaker, and they will not have the strength to pull the vertebra back.

The nervous system compensates by pulling in the opposite direction above and below the problem area. This creates a little zig zag in the spine. You might wonder whether moving two vertebrae out of place to deal with one displaced vertebra is such a good idea, however it is usually the best option that the nervous system has. Over a relatively short period of time, the spine either returns to balance, or the zig zags repeat themselves up and down the spine.

It's possible that the spine will return to balance because the compensatory pull actually moves the displaced vertebra more toward the center, thereby lengthening the shorter muscles and shortening the longer muscles. This allows the normal balancing functions of the muscles and nervous system to work properly. However, if this doesn't work and the zig zag becomes relatively permanent, the nervous system has no choice but to compensate for the compensators; the vertebra adjacent to a displaced vertebra will be pulled in the opposite direction, and then the vertebra adjacent to that one will pull back the other way, etc.

When we work with the alignment of the spine, we will immediately check for a zigzag pattern of fullness and emptiness up and down the spine. We want to release all the full areas, not spendng too much time with any one spot. Along with this, we also need to be working to repattern the way the nervous system interacts with the back. This means that, about halfway through working with the back, we should ask the client to get up and walk for just half a minute.

THE BACK AND SACRUM: GENERAL BALANCING AND QI FLOW

I will be describing this section from the standpoint of working on someone else, because it is obviously difficult to work on your own back.

Remember to use the centered breathing technique as you are working on your client. Keep checking in to your breath, and imagine it is moving into the area you are working on. And keep checking how you are feeling. The way you feel reflects the relationship you are developing with the person's body, spirit, and nervous system, and any information you can gather will often prove invaluable. You can't do that if you are taking it personally.

To begin with, we want to relax the back and open up the Bladder meridian, which flows down the back and the back of the legs. Massage this whole area, and as you do take notice of where the back is full or empty on which sides, and what sort of layers there are. Do parts of the back feel like a solid sheet, or are there lumps and bands of tension? Remember that we want to work with the solid sheets (first layer) to start, then move to the bands (second layer), then the knots (third layer).

Massage the back of the leg, especially the back of the knee at B 40 (at the popliteal crease). This is a release point for the whole back; use it whenever you feel like the back isn't releasing well. Find it by bending the knee to 90 degrees (the foot straight up when the person is on their back) and find the deepest part of the pocket created. Don't press this point hard, as it is sensitive and has important nerves and arteries running through it. Because it is a control point, by opening it up the back will continue to release long after we have finished.

Next, go to the fullest area of the back and begin to release/disperse it. Most likely, it will be fuller on one side of the spine—don't work on the emptier side, even if it is fuller than the rest of the back. You want to balance the spine left to right first, before you balance between different areas. If there are several areas which all feel very full, no matter—you will discover which one releases more slowly relatively soon, and that will be the most important area in the long run.

Spend some time as well balancing the pelvis. Look for which side of the pelvis is fuller at the top of the iliac crest (the gluteus medius and minimus) and then outside the bottom of the sacrum by the sitz bones (the ischial tuberosities, the bones you sit on) in the area of the gluteus maximus and piriformus muscles. Very often, you will find more fullness on the upper right and lower left.

There are certain warnings that you have worked long enough, starting with how you feel. The minute you feel bored, impatient, frustrated, or insecure, you need to evaluate the area. If it isn't feeling like it is releasing well, try approaching it differently. Try a different finger or a different angle, try to picture it more clearly. If it still doesn't change, move to another area of the back. In your mind's eye, step back and evaluate the whole back again. Go to the area which calls to you the most now, which feels fullest or the most impenetrable. Remember not to mistake bone for fullness; fullness has no detail and you cannot feel its depth; bone has detailed bumps and smooth spots, and you will be able to tell exactly how deep it is.

LOCATING THE SHU POINTS

As you release the back through each of the three layers, you will notice the individual Shu points emerging. You can determine which Shu points you are finding by reviewing the chart in Chapter 4 and the descriptions of the individual Shu point locations in each meridian chapter, and by checking individual point locations in Appendix A.

The Shu points extend from the upper thoracic area just below the shoulders to the bottom of the sacrum. Each of the Shu points will be two fingers out from the space between the spinous processes (the bump you feel on the back of each vertebra) except for the four Shu points of the sacrum. Remember that there is another set of Bladder points two fingers outside the regular Shu points, which we call the Outer Shu points. You won't be able to release the inner Shu's effectively until you release the outer Shu's.

THE SACROILIAC JOINT AND PELVIS

The pelvis can be difficult to visualize because it is a very three-dimensional structure, with movement in all three directions. There are three joints in the pelvis: two sacroiliac joints (or SI joints) on either side of the sacrum and the pubic symphysis, in the center of the pubic bone in the front. (A symphysis is a joint where two bones are joined together by cartilage.) The two sacroiliac joints are to the outside of the upper half of the sacrum, starting just inside the PSIS (the bump at the lower inside of the iliac crest) and the bottom of the joint is down about two inches from there.

The proper movement of the pelvis is dependent on the balance of the muscles, tendons and ligaments in this area. If there is a muscle which is tighter, or a ligament which is shorter, it will cause the pelvis to move differently. The lack of movement in one place created by tension or restriction will cause excessive movement in another area, and with excessive movement there is often irritation.

The most common pattern of imbalance with the pelvis is a torque pattern. With a healthy sacroiliac joint, the two hip bones will move in even opposition to each other as the person is walking. When the right leg goes forward, the right hip bone twists so that the top moves back and the bottom moves forward, and the left hip moves in the opposite direction (top forward and bottom back) because the left leg is moving backward. If the pelvis gets stuck at the end of this movement, the sacroiliac joint no longer moves as it should. The most common dysfunction is the pattern of the upper right coxal bone (the combination of the ileum, ischium and pubic bones) moved back and the lower right moved forward, and the opposite on the left side. We call this the standard torque, and it is almost universal.

So our job with the pelvis is to balance the tension and release/disperse areas of congestion and inflammation; front, back and sides. The most important area is the back of the pelvis, in the gluteal areas and the sacroiliac joint. Here, we will release/disperse the fullest areas, then release the ligamental and deep muscular support, then release/disperse the sacroiliac joint itself.

Start by checking to see which sides are fuller. Find the PSIS, the bump on the base of the iliac crest where it meets the sacrum. Check the entire muscular area outside the PSIS, anywhere within about three inches lateral of the PSIS, comparing both sides to see which is fuller. Also, release straight out to the side of the hip on the fuller side. Almost always, the right side is fuller, corresponding to the standard torque.

Now check in the piriformus area. Find the sitz bone, the ischial tuberosity, about three fingers beside and six fingers below the bottom of the sacrum. Compare the area between the ischial tuberosity and the bottom corner of the sacrum on both sides to feel which is the fullest. You will probably need to release cross-fiber, meaning to release across the muscle fibers stretching between the two points. If there is acute inflammation, you will need to disperse the area. Again, the most common pattern (the standard torque) is to have the lower left side tighter than the right.

The standard torque is an extremely common pattern with most people. Occasionally, someone will have more fullness on the upper left and lower right, occuring most commonly when the person has been in an accident or if they have been sitting for a long time in a bad chair. In this case, you will find that it usually straightens out very quickly and that it will often actually move back to a standard torque, which you will then have to treat.

Once you feel that the upper and lower sacroiliac joint area is relatively balanced (remember, we don't need to make it perfect, we need to initiate the release), we also need to release the front of the pelvis. This can make a huge difference with sacroiliac joint pain, because releasing excessive tension in the front will get rid of a lot of hypermobility in the SI joint.

Most commonly with the standard torque, the left inguinal area between the corner of the pubic bone and the ASIS is tighter. (The Anterior Superior Iliac Spine, or ASIS, is located at the top outside front of the hip). This is in the area of Sp 12 and 13. This is a sensitive area for most people, so be

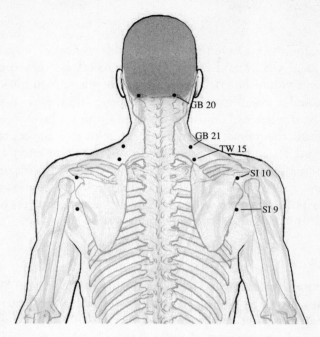

GB 20

GB 21

TW 15

SI 10

SI 9

SHOULDER AND NECK RELEASE

gentle. If they are ticklish, have them put their hand on top of your hand and this should greatly improve it.

Finish by massaging the hips and buttocks and down the legs.

RELEASING THE SHOULDER AND NECK

The neck and shoulders protect and enclose the spinal cord, which is the central organ of the nervous system. Many people hold tension here, and it is the source of most headaches and sinus and gland problems. Blockage in this area disrupts the central nervous system and may cause a lack of clarity, memory loss, mood problems, and any number of organ problems.

The shoulder and neck release is a technique that will relieve most people suffering from congestion in this area. I strongly suggest that you use it in every treatment, because blockage in this area is so common and so problematic.

To begin, have your client lie down on her stomach and approach from above the head.

THE POINTS

Five main acupoints are involved in the shoulder and neck release, SI 9 and 10, TW 15, and GB 21 and 20. If you were to release these points alone, your treatment would be effective, but not complete. You also release the neck and shoulder muscles once you have opened up the five points—these will act as "storm drains," allowing blocked Qi to drain.

After locating the points, it is important to release them accurately. Small Intestine 9 and 10 and TW 15 work to draw stagnant energy out of the shoulders long after you have released them. Gall Bladder 21, at the top of the shoulders, and GB 20, at the base of the skull, are commonly blocked points, corresponding to stress on the nervous system or stress on the body from external forces such as weather and exertion.

SI 9

Small Intestine 9 is located just behind the top of the armpit. You can find this point on yourself by putting your thumb into the armpit and your index finger behind the armpit and pinch; your finger will be close to SI 9. From there, simply feel for the outer edge of the scapula (shoulder blade). Slide up on the bone until you feel a muscle above your finger extending from the scapula to the arm—this is the teres muscle. Stay just below the teres and press into the edge of the scapula. You should feel a very precise area, about the size of a dime, which is painful; if not, move up and down the edge of the scapula until you do. Use a combination of deep, direct release and circular dispersal, then disperse the whole area.

SI 10

Small Intestine 10 releases Qi trapped in the shoulders, and once released continues to clear tension from the shoulders and neck.

Small Intestine 10 is located three fingers above SI 9. Trace a line from the back of the armpit up to the bony ridge, the spine of the scapula. Just below the spine of the scapula, feel for a sore spot not much bigger than SI 9, about half a finger-width (one finger-length being the width of the last segment of your index finger) below the spine. Slide left and right just below the spine until you feel it.

Use a deep, circular release, then disperse the whole area down through SI 9. After you have done both SI 9 and SI 10, work on the other side.

TW 15

This point is often called the "cold point," because it tends to become very tight and sore with a knot the size of a quarter at the onset of a cold or flu. Releasing this point frequently helps to prevent a cold.

Triple Warmer 15 is located on the top inside corner of the scapula, four fingers out from the spine and about three fingers below the top of the shoulder. Follow up the inside edge of the scapula (at the vertebral border) until you reach the top, then slide just up onto the top.

This point usually responds best to a combination of direct pressure release and circular dispersal.

GB 21

We call this point the "Weight of the World," or the "responsibility point." It gets tight when there is a lot of nervous system stress. It can also become congested at the onset of a cold or flu. This entire area may be congested and can be quite painful.

Find Gall Bladder 21 by locating the highest point of the shoulder, where it meets the side of the neck. From here, move toward the shoulder joint one finger. Massage the area to circulate Qi (cross-fiber massage, repeatedly moving from front to back to front with all four fingers, works great), and use direct pressure to release and disperse the point.

GB 20

This is the "back burner" point, a place we store tension from somewhere else. This point tends to get tight when you have a lot on your mind, but it can also be a place where "external wind"—cold wind or a draft on your neck—enters and causes your neck to become stiff or sore. This "wind" will move into the rest of the body, causing headaches, lung congestion, and deep pain in the back or arms. Gall Bladder 20 is located outside of the trapezius attachment on the back of the skull. Find the point where the trapezius attaches by following up the neck one finger outside the spine— you will feel cords under your fingers; this is the highest part of the trapezius. Follow it up until it ends in a bump on the skull. This is GB 20.

Release by using deep, steady release followed by circular dispersal. End by massaging the entire area down through the shoulders.

THE SHOULDER JOINT

Once you have released the shoulder points, you can then address the structure of the shoulder. The shoulder joint is composed of the upper arm bone (the humerus) and the glenoid cavity, a concave depression on the side of the scapula bone. It is a ball-and-socket joint. If you examine the bony structure of the joint, you can see that the ball of the humerus is held in the glenoid cavity by soft tissue; there is very little bone support.

The shoulder's movement is supported by both the clavicle and the scapula. The clavicle acts as a stabilizing bar, levering between the sternum and the acromion process, the bone at the top of the shoulder, a little toward the end. You can feel this by placing your right hand on your own left clavicle and then moving your arm directly above your head, and then directly out, away from your body, and then down, directly in front of your body. The clavicle itself is able to glide in all directions as you move your arm. Since the shoulder joint is on the end of the scapula, this allows movement of the arm—and the stress of its weight—to be spread over a wider area.

One thing you can do for shoulder problems, therefore, is to educate yourself and your client about the proper movement of the shoulder. A good exercise is to pretend that you are moving the joint from the center of the sternum, rather than from the shoulder joint alone. Put your left palm on the right side of your chest, with the heel of your hand at the sternum and the tips of your fingers at the shoulder joint. Extend your arm to the side and move your arm back and forth while keeping the shoulder joint relatively immobile. This should find you moving your arm and chest together, as if they were a single unit, rather than from the shoulder joint alone. (If you move the shoulder joint alone, it will protrude from the chest.) By moving the shoulder and chest together, the shoulder joint is supported.

Most shoulder joint problems stem from imbalances in the muscular support of the area. If there is excessive tension in the front of the joint, caused when the pectoral muscles are too tight, then the joint may partially dislocate forward. Even if this is not the case, imbalances in the joint support can cause limited range of motion that, over time, can worsen. Very often, such imbalances can manifest as hypermobility at the front of the joint and also at the back of the joint.

Hypermobility causes irritation of muscles, nerves, and bones. Several of the main nerves of the arm must pass over the front of the shoulder joint, and these can become irritated as well, leading to imbalances of the arm and hand. Such imbalances can give rise to chronic conditions, such as numbness, pain, weakness, or poor circulation. This can also be the beginning of conditions such as carpal tunnel syndrome or arthritis.

There are several possible causes of shoulder joint disorders. The main source is normal wear and tear that occurs from overwork or injury. Overwork can especially irritate the nerves. The shoulder can be thrown out of balance by nerve irritation originating in the neck, which itself arises from imbalances in the spine.

The nerves going to the arm originate from vertebrae C5 through T1. These nerves exit from the lower cervical spine and then interconnect with each other to form the brachial plexus. These nerves continue to form the four main nerves of the arm—the ulnar, median, radial, and musculocutaneous nerves—which innervate the entire shoulder girdle. If any of the lower cervical nerves of the spine become irritated and inflamed, the nerves in the arms can be affected, which in turn can disturb the balance and alignment of the shoulder. Of course, the reverse is possible as well: irritation of the shoulder nerves can inflame back pain and irritate the brachial plexus, affecting a wider area.

We can balance the spinal cervical nerves through the shoulder and neck release. When working on a person with shoulder or arm problems, do the shoulder release in conjunction with your work on the arms.

Our approach to shoulder imbalances is to release and balance the muscular support of the area; to release and disperse the exterior joint; and then to release and disperse inside the joint.

The muscular support for the "shoulder girdle" extends all the way from the top of the spine to the bottom of the thoracic vertebrae. We can break down our approach into releasing and balancing the muscles that move the scapula, the clavicle, and the humerus.

Start by feeling the entire shoulder girdle area, from just inside the scapula (on the back) and the sternum-pectoral area in the front out to the shoulder joint. Also, massage the top of the shoulder up to the neck. Feel for fullness and emptiness. Release the full areas to balance the joint. Pay special attention to releasing the pectoral muscles in the front of the chest— the pectoralis minor and major—to allow free movement but also to reduce any forward pull on the joint.

Also, after you have released the muscles, pull each shoulder back by sliding your hand under the scapula and dragging it downward and inward. At the same time, roll the shoulder itself backward and downward. This will extend and stretch the pectoral area, making it easier to release. By stretching the shoulder in this way—it is the opposite of a "hunched" back—you are helping to train the person in the proper positioning of the shoulder. After you have released the upper part of the chest, pull the shoulders back farther and release a little more.

Next, move to the shoulder joint itself. The joint capsule extends from the attachment at the scapula to just past the widest part of the ball of the humerus. Gently release and disperse this area, taking special care not to irritate the front of the joint. One of the best ways of working with this area is to hold the person's arm slightly forward (you can do this by grasping the arm with your closest arm and cradling it with your forearm and hip) while rubbing with the tips of your fingers on the front of the joint. As you massage, move your finger from an inward position—as if all the fingertips were close or touching—to an outward position, as if you were fanning your fingers outward.

Also, release the back of the joint. When the shoulder is slightly out of joint, muscles and ligaments tend to fill in the joint. By releasing the tension here, the shoulder is able to reseat itself in the joint. Work deeply and release the entire back shoulder area to a point about two fingers' distance below the scapula.

Next, use the ball of the humerus to release the joint. Grasp the shoulder joint with your near hand and the elbow with your other hand, cradling the forearm on your forearm and hip, and use the humerus to gently "stir" inside the joint. Go through a full circle motion in the joint several times in each direction, using the ball of the humerus to feel for any obstructions or tension. Feel especially in the back of the joint, as this is where more tension and obstruction tends to be. Massage it out with the head of the humerus. At the same time, you can use the fingers of your near hand to massage the different areas of the joint.

Lastly, we want to do a technique which tends to reseat the joint, yet is very gentle and safe. With the arm held the same way, gently pull downward (inferiorly) on the arm—apply only gentle and moderate pressure— as though you were pulling it slightly out of the joint. Hold for anywhere from five to ten seconds. Wait to feel a release, which will feel like a softening of the area. You may possibly feel the ball of the humerus drifting slightly down from the joint. As you gently pull, massage the joint with the fingers of your near hand, feeling for full areas and constriction. Rotate the humerus back (posteriorly) and sweep it up (superiorly) as it reaches its comfortable limit of movement. Massage the joint again with the head of the humerus.

You can determine the effects of this technique by comparing the two shoulders. The humerus of the shoulder not yet worked on, very often will jut forward of the joint, whereas the released shoulder is even with the joint. It is helpful to check both shoulder joints before you work on them. Once you know what to feel and look for, it will be easy to recognize this problem.

THE ELBOW JOINT

The cause of most elbow problems is a long-term imbalance between the inner and outer joint. Usually, the inside (medial) joint is excessively tight, causing hypermobility of the lateral joint which, over time, causes wear and tear. This is the classic "tennis elbow" syndrome. Again, this imbalance is almost always caused by irritation of the nerves in the neck.

To test for an imbalance between the two sides, grasp the arm, palm up, just above the elbow joint (toward the shoulder), while your other hand grasps the arm at the wrist. Lock the joint by bending the arm straight out, then unlock it slightly enough so you can feel some free play. Very gently rock the arm so that the forearm and upper arm move in opposite directions. This movement will cause the bones of the arm to rock across the elbow joint. You'll be able to determine if there is much mobility within the elbow joint.

If the joint is balanced, you will feel it lock into place at both ends of the movement, creating the sensation of what feels like a "thunk" at both ends of its movement. The joint has some mobility on both sides, but it is also able to lock into place as well. If, on the other hand, it is imbalanced, you will feel a distinct lock on one side of the joint—as if it is locked into place—but not on the other side. The loose side will feel as if the joint is stretching. When the joint is imbalanced, the side that stretches is hypermobile (it has too much movement in it), while the side that hinges is hypomobile (it has too little movement).

To help visualize this, imagine you have two blocks of wood butted against each other. Imagine you put the tip of a stick in between the two blocks, right in the middle, and then rock the two blocks against each other over the stick. You would feel the two blocks "clunk" together when they reached each other. Now, if you moved the stick more to one side of the "joint," and then rock the blocks, they will only "clunk" on one side. The side of the elbow joint that is too tight is like the side with the stick in it; it will act as a hinge.

This "hinge," or hypomobile side, is most commonly on the inside of the arm—the part closest to the body—and is caused by excessive fullness along the Heart Meridian, which is also the path of the ulnar nerve. As you know, excessive stress affects the heart and heart meridian. Heart 3 is located at the medial elbow joint and is an excellent indicator for long-term stress if it is tightly knotted.

To release the point, use a gentle releasing pattern in the direction of the meridian, rather than cross fiber. Apply gentle pressure and wait patiently for the point to release. If you can initiate this sort of gentle release, the point will continue to release over time; you will not have to keep massaging the point once it releases. Once you release the point, rub lightly with the tips of your fingers up and down the heart meridian, from just below the armpit to the pinky finger, along the inside of the arm.

If the other side of the elbow is hinging, it means the lung meridian (especially Lu 5) is imbalanced. Release Lu 5 in the same way. Release the muscles of the joint from the upper arm just below the shoulder joint all the way to below the elbow. Feel for fullness and emptiness in a neutral position, then gently twist the forearm to its comfortable extremes in both directions, feeling for fullness and emptiness at either extreme. Release any fullness you perceive.

Next, release and disperse the joint itself. If you have already released Ht 3 or Lu 5, you have already started. The joint area surrounds the joint itself, extending about one finger's distance both above and below the joint. Using the flat of the tips of your fingers, look for knots of congestion, and be careful not to irritate the ulnar nerve both at Ht 3 and SI 8, just midway to the point of the elbow (the olecranon process).

Lastly, clear the inside of the joint. This can be done by releasing and dispersing at the joint itself. Gently release the hypomobile side, massaging gently around the ulnar nerve area. Release any knots around the hyper-mobile side. Finish by massaging the whole joint area.

THE WRIST AND FOREARM

Wrist problems are most commonly caused by excessive tension in the flexors, the muscles in the inner forearm which flex the wrist and bend the fingers. Typically, the flexors will have tension, while the extensors on the other side are inflamed from overuse. This imbalance in the flexors can be caused by nerve irritation which can cause tension in the muscles directly affected by the nerve, but it can also be caused by excessive use.

A classic cause of excessive flexor tension is typing or playing piano, where there is much more effort to push down with the fingers and hands, and hence more exercise for the flexors. It is also positional—by using the flexors while the palms are in the down position (pronation) with the wrists hyperextended. This is a relatively unnatural posture, compared to most things we do with our hands.

Typically, this posture causes the anterior forearm and flexors to become full and the posterior forearm and extensors (which pull the wrist and fingers back) comparatively empty. In addition, the pronators (which rotate the hand inward) are full and the supinators (which rotate the hand outward) are empty.

To begin the release, massage the forearm to release the full areas. Extend the wrist but just until the flexors become taut, not to their extreme, and release the flexors. Turn the hand to twist the forearm in both directions, releasing the fullest muscles in each position. Remember, when releasing, apply pressure and wait for the area to release. You want to work the area like cold clay, to warm it up and increase its mobility and blood flow.

Also, spend some time releasing the interosseous membrane, the band of ligament between the radius and the ulna. To do this, release along the pericardium and Triple Warmer meridians, on the front and back of the midline of the forearm, while pronating and supinating (twisting) the forearm. You especially want to release this area with the forearm in the palms-up position (supinated).

Next, release the wrist and palm. You can think of the wrist as made up of three joints: one at the wrist where the radius and ulna of the forearm meet the first row of carpal bones in the hand; the next about a finger-width away, or distal (toward the fingers), where the first row of carpal bones meets the second; and a third, one finger distal to that, where the second row of carpal bones meets the metacarpals. In addition to these movements, the hands have to move so that the palms can close, such as when the thumb and pinky touch each other.

All of these bones need to move freely. Any lack of mobility, which is caused by fullness, will create excessive mobility—or emptiness—in another area of the hand or wrist. Go through the wrist and the first half of the palm (the carpal bones) to feel for any bones which seem hard or inflexible. As you find them, spend some time releasing the muscles and tissues around them, especially on the full side (usually the palm side). Again, work the area like cold clay as you release; try to move the particular bones which feel stiffer toward the full side.

Next, release the joints. Each space between a bone is a joint. We want all of the joints to be equally mobile, so spend most of your time releasing the joints between bones which don't want to move. Again, think of releasing the deep joint as releasing a chronic "plug," then release and disperse under the plug. Go back and forth between releasing the tissues around the bones and releasing the joints. End with deep massage of the wrist, palm, and forearm.

THE HAND AND FINGERS

We've already released most of the palm of the hand, now let's release the rest. One way of seeing the hand is to see the fingers as extending all the way to the third wrist joint, or all the way to the metacarpal bones. Indeed, if you were looking at a skeleton and had no idea what the creature's flesh looked like, you would see the fingers as much longer than they look from the outside. Most of the articulation we have in our fingers comes more from the phalanges, the three bones of the fingers, but the metacarpals do contribute some movement.

First, let's spend some time releasing between the metacarpals. We have worked with the Large Intestine 4 area (LI 4) in the thick muscle between the thumb and first finger. Massage this point deeply, releasing the point and the whole muscle itself.

Check out the movement of the thumb and finger, and how they affect this area. Now go through each of the other spaces between metacarpal bones, sliding the bones to articulate each in relation to the adjacent bones. Perhaps the best way to release these spaces is to come from between the fingers and use your index finger and thumb as a pincer to massage the space.

Next, let's release each of the finger joints. First, massage the joint and the area around it. Evaluate its movement, flexing and extending each joint as you massage it. See if the tendons move freely and feel evenly full, without any empty or thinner spots. If you find a thinner area of a tendon, spend some time releasing the full areas.

Check to see if there is excessive mobility to either side of the joint, or excessive congestion on one side that might prevent the joint from settling on that side. Release the more congested side (the hinge, just as we did with the elbow). Then release and disperse in the joint space itself. Look for knots of congestion preventing inflammation from escaping from the deep joint, and clear them before releasing and dispersing the joint.

End by massaging the hand and fingers.

Remember to massage the entire area—from the shoulders to the tips of the fingers—gently and firmly. Probe intelligently with your fingers, assessing each and every place you work on. This requires concentration and continual assessment of the points, meridians, tissues, and joints. Once you have applied your skill and released the shoulders, arms, elbows, wrists, palms, and fingers, the person you have worked on will feel tremendous relief and relaxation in the upper part of his or her body. The Qi will now be flowing along all the relating meridians and healing their respective organs.

RELEASING THE LEGS

Once you have released the shoulders and neck move to the opposite end of the body and release the foot, calf, knee and hip joint.

ABOUT THE FOOT AND CALF

The Integrative Acupressure approach to the foot is to return it to normal functioning. The foot can be seen as an elongated tripod, with the heel being the main weight-bearing leg and the other two legs, the pad, acting to stabilize the foot. When we look at the bones of the foot, we can see that the first three toes, along with the cuneiform and talus bones, act together, as do the fourth and fifth toes along with the cuboid and the calcaneus, or heel bone.

Functionally, it's as though there were actually two long toes, one starting higher up on the ankle and going to the inside of the foot, and one starting at the bottom of the heel and going to the outside of the foot. If the foot is out of balance, these two "toes" will be out of balance with each other. If the medial (inner)"toe" is weak, the lateral (outer) "toe" will have to compensate for it by taking on the majority of the support. With the balance of the foot off, the knee, hip, and spine, as well as the whole body, are affected.

There is also an intimate relationship between the medial toe and the tibia, the inner bone of the calf, and the lateral toe and the fibula, the smaller outer bone of the calf. When we invert, or tilt the foot inward as though we were walking sideways on a hill, the tibia must move forward and the fibula back, rotating around each other. When we evert, or tilt the foot outward, the fibula must move forward and the tibia back.

If the foot is imbalanced and the tibia and fibula aren't able to move freely, this will throw off the foot's ability to balance. You will then have either pronation (the foot collapses inward when walking) or supination (walking on the outside of the foot). A quick way of diagnosing this is to check your shoes. If the sole of the shoe is wearing more toward the inside, this is an indication of pronation. If the shoe is wearing on the outside edge, this indicates supination. If it is wearing on an angle from the heel, this shows external rotation of the foot (splayed).

When working to balance the foot, start with the heel, then balance the pad, then ensure that the entire foot is working together. The idea is to allow the foot to comfortably adapt to whatever terrain we are walking on. Our ancestors walked either barefoot or with very thin, flexible shoes so their feet could adapt this way. Because of the way the foot is designed, the heel supports most of the weight and the pad balances the foot and the whole body. The heel is relatively pointed; it is not designed to balance, any more than the heel of a high-heeled shoe is designed to balance.

The foot is designed to balance the body by twisting the pad in relation to the heel. This allows the pad of the foot to do its job of adapting to the terrain while the heel supports most of the weight. However, when we wear shoes, this prevents the heel and foot from working independently. As a consequence, the muscles that support the pad become more rigid and the muscles that normally stabilize the heel adapt. The heel, which normally is a relative point, becomes functionally much wider. Hence, the heel adapts to support and balance the foot.

The muscles that support the heel, the tibialis posterior and peroneus longus, are long, relatively weak muscles that cannot support the foot as needed. Consequently, the foot becomes unstable and more prone to injuries like sprains. Along with this, the muscles of the lower leg are supported by the meridians passing through them. When these meridians are imbalanced, the muscles also become imbalanced. Look for such an imbalance; it manifests in the way the feet are held and the way they move, especially in the way a person compensates for imbalanced terrain.

RELEASING THE FOOT

When working with the feet, it may seem easiest to work from below, facing the bottom of the feet. However, this forces you to use your thumbs. It is very important to be careful when using your thumbs, so it's best if you can minimize their use. For this reason, you should work with the client's leg at your side, facing the top of the foot. This also allows you to stabilize the leg while you work.

You need to balance the heel first. Usually, there is excessive tension inside the heel just below and behind the anklebone, or medial malleolus. This pulls the heel inward. With your own foot, try feeling for tension in this area. Pull the area tight by pulling outward laterally on the heel with one hand and feel for bands of tension between the medial malleolus and the back and bottom of the heel. There are usually three places, or three bands, where tension can occur. Starting at the bottom of the medial malleolus, find the middle band, which runs diagonally down toward the heel. The posterior band is just above this, starting at the same point below the malleolus and extending back horizontally and slightly downward. If this band is tight, it will cause the foot to splay outward. The inferior band starts at the same point and extends downward and slightly back. This band will cause the heel to invert and the person will either walk on the outside of the foot or collapse through the arch.

These bands are easily released by massaging the tightest band while pulling the heel out, in order to stretch the band at the same time. After a while, you will find that this band is no longer the tightest of the three; at this point, find the next tightest band and do the same massage until it is also loose. By now, the heel should be relatively loose.

Now check beneath the outside anklebone, the lateral malleolus. You will find that directly below the lateral malleolus and extending back, there is a joint between the talus above and calcaneus below. This is the subtalar joint. If the vertical band was the tightest, there would be an area of congestion directly below the lateral malleolus. If the diagonal band was the tightest, the area of congestion would be slightly behind this point, about a finger's distance. One finger behind that, just below and forward from the attachment of the Achilles tendon, would be congested if the horizontal band was the tightest. These areas would be painful on pressure; massage the tightest point until it dissipates.

The reason these points get so tight is because the tension below the medial malleolus closes the joint on that side and opens the joint on the lateral side. When a joint is too tight on one side and too lose on the other, it causes the joint to be hypermobile, or too movable, on the side that is excessively open. This excessive movement creates irritation and inflammation; the knots you feel are the result, and, like a doorstop, they prevent the joint from closing on that side. Because of this, the heel is always slightly inverted. By releasing these knots, you are allowing proper alignment of the heel.

Once the heel is balanced, you need to balance the pad, or forefoot. The two most common imbalances of the pad are excessive tension under the lateral, or outside edge, of the mid foot and excessive tension of the tibialis anterior muscle, which attaches halfway up the arch, and serves to lift the inner foot and first, second, and third toes. The origin of the tibialis anterior is on the front outside of the shin just below the kneecap. It crosses the tibia (shinbone) just above the ankle. Most of this is running along the stomach meridian, to the outside of the tibia.

You need to evaluate which of these two imbalances is predominant. To do this, grasp the heel with one hand and stabilize it while twisting the pad with the other. Most people's feet invert, or flex so that the inside moves up and the outside moves down, very well. Eversion, on the other hand, is usually somewhat limited. When you try to twist the foot so that the big toe moves down and the pinky toe moves up, you will probably find that there is relatively limited motion. Whichever side moves the least is the side you want to release.

If the area under the lateral side (outer side) of the foot is the tightest, deeply massage the soft area between the pad and the heel on the outside of the foot. This is in the area of the fourth and fifth metatarsal bones. As you release the area, make sure that the bones are moving freely. By mobilizing the bones at the same time you massage the area, you can increase the effectiveness of the release.

If the predominant imbalance is excessive tension in the inner foot, we need to release above the arch, following up the tendon of the tibialis anterior to just below the knee. This area, from where the tendon crosses the tibia up to the outer knee, is the path of the stomach meridian. Massage this area deeply, first across the muscle fibers then in the direction of the muscle. Notice that the tightest areas are usually just below the knee (Stomach 36) and halfway between the ankle and knee (Stomach 40). Follow the path of the tendon, massaging across the tendon somewhat gently while you plantarflex the foot downward.

Once you have balanced the heel and pad, you need to work with the whole foot. It's best if you can sit right next to the client's knee, with her leg on top of your lower thigh so that you can grasp her shin firmly. Place your forearm on top of her shinbone with your elbow near her knee, and hold the ankle just above the malleoli. Grasp the pad with your other hand and begin to rotate the foot. You want the foot to rotate such that the toe draws a circle in the air. While you are doing this, make sure that the pad stays perpendicular to the leg: Don't allow the inner or outer foot to move upward or downward. Imagine that you are keeping the pad even with an imaginary floor. If you are doing it properly, the pad will twist in relation to the heel as you rotate.

What you will notice is that the toe does not trace a perfect circle; certain parts of the circle will be somewhat flattened because of tension in the foot, ankle, and calf. It is relatively easy to see that tension in the back of the leg prevents the foot from being able to dorsiflex upward adequately, and excessive tension in the front will prevent the foot from plantarflexing downward well. What is less easy to see is what prevents other motions. Remember, in order for the foot to move in a certain direction, something must stretch. The tightest area of the ankle, when you turn the foot in a circular motion, is the area you want to work on.

Imagine that the circle that the right toe traces is a clock, with 12:00 being upward (dorsiflexion) and 6:00 being downward (plantarflexion). If the right foot cannot move well toward 3:00 (to the right), there is excessive tension below the medial malleolus. If it cannot move well toward 4:00, there is tension just in front of the medial malleolus. If the foot cannot move well toward 9:00 (to the left), there is tension below the lateral malleolus; similarly, tension just behind the lateral malleolus will prevent the toe from moving fully toward 10:00.

Release accordingly, then spend some time with the foot after these three releases. Look for areas of tension, congestion, or lack of movement, especially in the area of the metatarsals in the mid foot.

BALANCING THE TIBIA AND FIBULA

As I said before, when we invert and evert the foot (turn it inward and outward), this causes the tibia and fibula to rotate around each other. When the foot inverts, the tibia moves forward and the fibula moves back; similarly, when we evert the foot, the tibia moves back and the fibula moves forward.

Try this for yourself. Cross your right leg with the upper ankle over the left knee. Hold your ankle just above the malleoli with your right hand and hold the foot with the left hand and invert it, tilting the heel and toe toward the ceiling, then evert it, tilting the whole foot toward the floor. Notice how the ankle must twist as you do this. Now try twisting the ankle at the same time. As you invert the foot, twist so that the inside of the ankle (facing up) is moving forward and the outside (facing down) is moving back, then the opposite way as you evert.

This will probably take a few tries, because you are having to do two things at once. If you can't distinctly feel how your tibia and fibula are rotating, try twisting the opposite way; inward as you evert and outward as you invert. You should feel much more resistance to the twisting motion.

If there is congestion or muscular tension preventing proper movement of the tibia and fibula, the foot won't be able to move properly. Most often, the tibia is held slightly anterior to the fibula, causing a tendency to invert the foot. Because of this, you might think that most people would pronate, or walk on the outside of the foot, but usually people compensate by externally rotating, or splaying the feet outward (duck-foot) or by collapsing through the arch. You can tell when someone has this problem because the heel is bent inward significantly.

To release this, we must release the area around the interosseous membrane (*interosseous* means "between bone"), the tissue between the tibia and fibula, running the length of the shin. With your fingers in back of the calf and thumb in front, find the outer edge of the tibia in the front and back and move outward from here. Your fingers should be squeezing toward your thumb, into the space between the tibia and fibula. Massage up and down this area until you find the tightest spot; usually this is about halfway up the calf in the front—at Stomach 40. This is a point for excess dampness, or mucus, in the digestive system. Another common area of tension is in the upper calf, at Stomach 36, which is a tonifying, or building, point for the digestive system and for the energy of the whole body. It's one of the most powerful points in acupressure.

Massage this area deeply with one hand while grasping the upper foot. You can increase the release by rotating the tibia and fibula around each other. Do this by alternately inverting and everting the foot. You can increase the effect of this by twisting the calf at the same time—twist so that the tibia moves forward as the foot inverts, then twist so that the fibula moves forward as the foot everts. This takes a bit of practice to master; you want to get to the point where you can massage at the same time that you are rotating the tibia and fibula. Massage the entire interosseous area from the ankle to below the knee until the area feels looser. Remember that the area will continue to loosen over the next several days; don't try to make it perfect.

RELEASING THE KNEE

The knee is one of the most complicated joints of the body. Even so, we can make a remarkable difference in its functioning. Most knee problems result from long-term imbalances in the feet or the muscles of the upper leg and hips. As we have addressed imbalances in the feet, we will be covering hip imbalances next.

For the knees, we need to release the muscles that support and balance the knee.

First, feel the thigh for imbalances in muscular tone. Obviously, the outer thigh is less muscular than the inner, and the front quadriceps are not as strong as the back hamstrings; we are looking for balanced tone, not muscle strength. Feel for areas of fullness and congestion. Start by releasing across the fibers, massaging to separate the muscles from each other.

You will often find that there is considerable fullness on the lower inner thigh, and even greater fullness on the upper outer thigh. This shows that the sartorius, the longest muscle in the body, is being used excessively. This muscle, also called the "tailor's muscle," is used to lift the foot up to cross the legs. It is not normally used in stabilization of the knee, but if the foot is pronating, the knee will tend to fall inward. The body will use this muscle to pull the knee back out again, and over time the muscle becomes over-developed. You will need to release the sartorius so that the nervous system will learn to compensate correctly. You can do this by massaging the muscle deeply.

RELEASING THE HIP JOINT

Many people find the hip joint intimidating because it's large, difficult to manipulate through so much tissue and large bone, and seemingly immov-able. Actually, it's not as tough as it might initially appear.

First, you need to know where the hip joint is, which may not be as evident as some may think. From the front of the hip, find the point halfway between the bump on the front corner of your hip (known as the anterior-superior iliac spine), and the corner of the pubic bone, just below the in-guinal ligament (Sp 13). The hip joint is located directly behind this. From the back, it is located two fingers outside and three fingers up from the sitz bone (the ischial tuberosity), or about five fingers outside the bottom of the sacrum where it meets the coccyx (GB 30).

Most people who are complaining of hip pain will point to the area directly on the side of the hip, where the top of the femur bone (the top of the thigh bone is known as the greater trochanter) joins with the hip. This is an attachment point for muscles that control the leg. Pain can radiate from the side of the hip, or along the lower back and then down the leg (following the sciatic nerve). The release I am going to describe will help people with a full range of hip, lower back problems, and pain that extends down the leg to the foot.

Your client should be lying on his or her back, preferably on a massage table, or the floor. (If you are working on yourself, lie on your back or sit on the floor or a bed with plenty of support.) Explore the entire hip area deeply, feeling for excessive fullness or for differences in fullness and emptiness. Check all sides of the upper thigh area, the outside hip, lower back along the hip line, and the front of the pelvis, the area around Sp 13. Release and disperse the fullness or congestion you encounter. Also, disperse any painful or acutely inflamed areas.

Next, we want to clear the synovial area around the hip joint. Start by releasing deeply in the area just above the greater trochanter (again, the top of the femur bone, where it joins the hip). Disperse the area if there is more inflammation. Because the joint is deep and well protected, you may have to work deeply into the tissue, even as you disperse the area. Remember to do this gently, but deeply. Move deliberately but with sensitivity, knowing that the area may be tender and painful to the client. Try to picture the joint. Also, picture the inflammation and any stagnation being released. Concentrate on releasing the entire area from Sp 13 to GB 30. Also release the area that is down about four fingers from GB 30.

Next, release inside the joint itself, which can be done by moving the leg to massage the joint where the ball of the femur bone sits inside the hip bone, or ischium. I'll describe the technique for the right leg. Simply reverse it for the left leg.

Start by grasping the leg about halfway down the calf with your right hand. With your left hand, grasp around the front and back of the hip at the greater trochanter. Lift the leg with both hands and begin moving the ball of the femur in the joint, as though you were stirring a big spoon inside the joint. This will help to clear the joint of stagnant Qi, resistance, and congestion. As you do this, you should be able to "feel" inside the joint for obstructions or excessive movement. (Practice and experience dealing with a variety of hip joints will allow you to be able to determine whether the joint is congested.)

If the leg is heavy and your arms are tired, use the side of your hip to support the leg and your right hand. You will need to move your whole body in order to rotate the leg, but the movement makes rotating a heavy leg much easier. If this still doesn't work, set the leg down and put your hands beneath the leg. Lift the leg while the backs of your hands are still on the table or bed. This will limit your movement significantly, but it is better than not working the joint at all.

Lastly, release the joint with the knee bent and the foot resting on the table. Grasp the hip joint with both hands, one in front and the other on the back, and gently move it up and down. Try to rotate the hip slightly and gently. The disadvantage to this technique is that you cannot move the joint very much. Also, this technique doesn't give you a clear assessment of the tightness or congestion of the hip because the ligaments tighten when the leg is straight and loosen significantly when the leg is bent. Thus, you won't be able to tell if the ligaments are too loose. You will be able to release some tension from the hip, however, which will be therapeutic.

Finish by massaging the entire joint area and the muscles.

COMPLETING THE TREATMENT

At this point, it is very helpful to massage the feet and lower legs, which draws the energy down from the head into the legs and feet, thus relieving pressure and tension that have accumulated in the upper body.

End by placing your palms on the lower abdomen and the top of the client's head. This activates and balances the flow of Qi between the head and bottom of the torso. It also harmonizes the nervous system. When you've spent a few moments holding the person in this way, the treatment is over.

This release alone will make many clients feel infinitely better about their bodies and their lives. It restores the flow of energy throughout the body and, in the process, gives back a sense of perspective on life. It's a good way to finish a treatment.

Acupressure Lymphatic Release

Acupressure Lymphatic Release (ALR) cleanses the lymph system of toxins that have been stored in the cells, tissue fluid, and organs, and thereby boosts the immune system. It is one of the most important and powerful methods of healing, especially for anyone with an immune or chronic disease, environmental illness, or some form of degenerative illness.

One of the more remarkable facts about the lymph system is that it is virtually ignored by Western medicine, yet is an essential system by which the body rids itself of poisons, pathogens, and cellular debris. A lymph system that is rife with environmental toxins, viruses, or bacteria is a breeding ground for disease. Therefore, one of the greatest things you, as an acupressure therapist, can do for your client is to promote movement and elimination of waste from the lymph system.

THE LYMPH: CLEANSING YOUR INNER SYSTEM

The lymphatic system is two and a half times as long as the cardiovascular system. This vast circulatory system runs from the bottoms of the feet to the top of the head. Yet it only runs in one direction—from the cells of your body to a pair of openings behind the clavicle bones, where it pours its waste into the bloodstream. The bloodstream carries the waste to the liver and kidneys to be neutralized and eliminated from the body.

As you probably already know, most of the body is actually water and most of that water surrounds cells and cellular material. The water is rich with oxygen, nutrition, immune cells, and antibodies. These substances virtually bathe the cells in all that they need to survive and even thrive. This water, also known as intercellular fluid or interstitial fluid, also contains the waste products from cells, including carbon dioxide and broken and dead cells, as well as many substances that are potentially disease-causing to humans, such as viruses, bacteria, and environmental toxins, some of which may be cancer-causing substances. Most immune battles are waged here, in the interstitial fluid, and in the bloodstream.

Much of the interstitial fluid (about 40 percent) returns to the blood by passing through the capillary walls, a process called osmosis. The remaining 60 percent passes into the capillaries and vessels of the lymph system, at which point interstitial fluid becomes lymph fluid. Among the waste products that become part of the lymph, and travel within the lymph system, are all nonsoluble particulate matter, such as carbon particles, dead cell debris, heavy metals, and many other environmental poisons.

Like a vast network of train tracks, lymph vessels traverse the entire body, entering and exiting every part of the body, including every tissue, organ, and system. One of the organs through which the lymph vessels pass is the small intestine, the organ that absorbs nutrients from food. Inside the small intestine are tiny fingerlike projections, called villi, that are nutrient-absorbing. Inside the villi are tiny blood capillaries, which allow nutrition to pass into the blood. Also in the villi are lymphatic capillaries, called lacteals, that absorb nutrients and fats into the lymph system, which also brings such nutrients to cells.

Among the organs of the lymph system are the lymph nodes. Lymph nodes act as filters of the lymph fluid, breaking down and removing disease-causing agents, including those that would cause infection. Lymph nodes also produce lymphocytes and monocytes, both important immune cells. Lymph nodes can be the size of a pinhead or as big as a lima bean. They are scattered throughout the body, with major clusters occurring in certain regions of the body; such clusters are called regional lymph nodes.

Three of these regional node clusters drain the extremities (legs, arms, neck, and head), and the skin and surface tissues of the body. They are located in the groin (inguinal nodes), which drain the tissues below the navel, including the legs; under the armpits (axillary nodes), which drain between the navel and the clavicles, including the arms; and around the jaw (cervical nodes), which drain the head and neck.

The entire lymph system brings the lymph to two exit points: the ends of the right lymphatic duct, behind the right clavicle bone, and the thoracic duct, behind the left. The lymph drains into the blood and is cleansed by the liver. The openings of these ducts are quite small, about half the size of a pencil. Therefore, it is very easy to cause the lymph system to back up if the ducts become partially closed, as they can be from a variety of causes, among which is the muscle tension we experience in our shoulders.

Numerous important organs are part of the lymph system, including the spleen, thymus, tonsils (including the "regular," or palatine, tonsils; the pharyngeal tonsils, also known as the adenoids; and the lingual tonsils which are little mounds of lymphoid tissue on the back of the tongue), and lymph nodes (which produce the lymphocytes and B-cells).

Pumping the Lymph System

Because the lymph system has no heart as the blood system does, the body as a whole must pump the lymph. This is accomplished in several ways, including the contraction and expansion of muscles, the movements of the diaphragm during respiration, bowel elimination, and the many involuntary movements that are part of human activity.

Inside the lymph vessels and capillaries are valves that allow lymph fluid to move only in the direction of the drainage points behind the clavicle bones. Because of these valves, any kind of compression of the body moves the lymph forward, toward the drainage sites.

Breathing and involuntary muscle action are inadequate by themselves to keep the lymph moving sufficiently over prolonged periods of time. Unless additional activity occurs, interstitial fluid collects in the lungs and other organs and tissues, creating a breeding ground for infection and pneumonia. Such stagnation of the lymph system can lead to an array of disorders, including the diminished flow of nutrients and oxygen to the cells; the buildup of toxins and debris in the tissues; and the reduced effectiveness of the immune system. A poorly functioning lymph system always leads to a poorly functioning body.

It is for this reason that hospital personnel routinely move bedridden patients several times a day—to get the lymph moving and prevent congestion and stagnation of lymph fluid.

Still, the more sedentary your lifestyle, the greater the danger of stagnating your lymph system and creating the basis for a wide array of illnesses. This is one of the reasons exercise is so important. During exercise, lymph flow increases by ten to fifteen times over that of resting flow.

The great majority of Americans do not get enough exercise, which puts many at risk. That's why acupressure lymphatic release is so important.

THE BENEFITS OF LYMPHATIC RELEASE

Acupressure lymphatic release optimizes the drainage of the lymph system by stimulating specific acupressure points that directly affect the circulation of lymph fluid and release of the major ducts, trunks, nodes, and capillaries of the lymph system.

We augment these steps by balancing the function of the spleen meridian, which governs the lymphatic system, and by applying direct pressure in specific locations to assist in the pumping of lymph.

If we increase the flow and drainage of lymph, all the functions related to the lymph system can be improved. So, too, can many conditions that are wholly or partially the result of lymphatic stagnation. Clients often tell me that after having their lymph systems regularly released, they experience relief of chronic colds and all signs related to a weakened immune system; allergies, chronic fatigue, environmental illnesses, and skin problems improve. So, too, do disorders of the breast and sinuses.

Dramatic improvements in health can occur when lymphatic release is combined with regular acupressure or acupuncture; improvements in diet and exercise patterns; and the use of other natural healing methods, such as homeopathy.

PREPARATION FOR ALR

A WORD OF CAUTION

Like all other powerful healing tools, acupressure lymphatic release must be used wisely and with some caution. Any technique that causes the discharge of toxins into the bloodstream or that stimulates the boosting of the immune system is, in itself, a stressor on the body. My experience has been that lymphatic work can sometimes cause unpleasant or even mildly debilitating side effects, such as headaches, flulike symptoms, and fatigue, if the blood-cleansing organs are not strong enough to handle the cellular discharge.

Consequently, I usually spend several treatment sessions strengthening the blood-cleansing and eliminative organs and their related meridians—namely, the liver, kidneys, bladder, lungs, and large intestine. Generally, I do not begin to work with the lymphatic system directly at least until the third session, and then it is only with healthy people. For those with long-standing health problems, I do not recommend using the lymphatic release until after they have experienced six to ten treatments, during which all the blood-cleansing and eliminative organs and meridians have been strengthened. Even then, I use the lymphatic release gently.

Acupressure lymphatic release should not be considered a replacement for the care of a licensed health professional when there is a possibility that a serious illness is present. Consult a medical doctor, homeopath, naturopath, chiropractor, acupuncturist, or some other health professional for any long-standing or chronic conditions.

Also, when you feel that your client is ready for a lymphatic release, do a very gentle version of it the first time, and then gradually increase the work as the client's condition improves. Each ALR session should include this preparatory release.

Preparatory Steps

Even before you begin working on the lymph system, it's important to prepare the client's body by boosting Qi flow to the elimination and blood-cleansing organs. To do this, follow these directions:

1. With the client on his stomach, release the spleen, liver, and kidney source points on the foot.

2. Massage the bladder meridian down the back and the back of the legs, including Bladder 40.

3. Release the Shu points on the back for kidney (small of the back, halfway between the hips and the ribs); spleen (three vertebrae above the kidney Shu); and liver (two vertebrae above the spleen Shu, or two down from the level of the bottom point of the scapula).

4. Have the person turn over and do the shoulder and neck release described in chapter 20.

5. Release the clavicle area. By releasing the clavicle area, you open the exit ducts and allow lymph to flow more smoothly throughout the system. If the clavicle ducts are not sufficiently open, the lymph in the upper chest backs up and stagnates.

    Massage beneath and above the clavicle bone from Kidney 27 past Stomach 12 and 13, and Lung 2 out to the end of the clavicle, paying special attention to both ends of the bone. The ends of the bone are usually the primary sites of tension, and often one will be tight while the other is loose. Your task is to try to even this difference by massaging the tighter side, whether it is the attachment to the sternum or the area by the shoulder.

Massage Technique: Like Combing Long Hair

When releasing the major ducts and vessels of the lymph system, one consideration you must constantly bear in mind is this: *You must always give the lymph fluid somewhere to go.* This may seem elementary, but it is the cornerstone of ALR and cannot be emphasized enough.

As I said earlier, the lymphatic ducts, trunks, and capillaries have millions of one-way valves in them, allowing the lymph only to move toward its eventual drainage site and back into the blood circulation. If you do not open the ducts, but work on the lymph system, you may irritate or injure the lymphatic organs, such as the lymph nodes.

Work on a person's lymph system as if you were combing very long hair. If you were to start combing at the top of the head, the comb would get caught in the tangle of hairs as you tried to slide the comb downward. Pretty soon, it would be snarled in knots. The best way to do the job is to start at the bottom of the hair, combing out only a few inches, but avoiding the snarls. As the hair straightens, you can move upward a few inches at a time until eventually you can slide the comb from the top of the head to the end of the hair. It's the same with the lymph system.

If you were to try to release the lymph by starting far away from the site of drainage (the clavicle area at the neck), you would be pressing against whatever accumulation of debris and tension there is in the whole system. There's too much resistance in the system for you to be able to start, say, at the toes or the fingers or even the arms. If you tried, you'd cause a ballooning of the lymphatic vessels where blockages are located.

The best approach is to *start at the drainage point—at the clavicle area— and work backward while pushing the lymph forward.* Think of the drainage point as being the ends of the hair. Start by releasing this area and then, a few inches at a time, move backward, always moving the lymph forward toward the drainage ducts.

As you work, your image of the lymph should be that of a viscous fluid. You aren't going to be able to push it fast. Instead, apply gentle but direct pressure on the exit points and the entire clavicle area; allow your fingers to sink directly into the tissue and then slide your fingers forward in the direction of the lymph flow. Apply pressure in such a way that you press downward, at first, and then move the lymph forward toward the exit points as you feel the lymph release. As stated earlier, even just compressing the lymph ducts will serve to squeeze the lymph along.

You will find that, as you progress through the ALR series, the lymphatic areas will feel less and less viscous and unyielding, and more and more soft and quick to release.

Look for the subtleties of the body's response to your pressure; notice the changes in the areas on which you are working, and in the body as a whole. As you become involved in the body's subtle interaction, you may notice more responses in your client that you once thought were "imaginary."

ACUPRESSURE LYMPHATIC RELEASE

After you have completed the preparatory work, ask your client to lie on his or her back on your massage table. Place yourself behind his or her head, so that you are looking downward at the client's face and then place the palms of your hands on each of the client's shoulders.

The first step will be to release the points that provide Qi to the drainage points behind the clavicle bones. These drainage points are located behind the clavicle, about halfway out from the point where the clavicle bones attach to the sternum at the neck and chest area. Put your four fingers on the clavicle with the index finger on the knob at the inner end of the bone, and then measure out four fingers' distance. Just above this point on the clavicle is Stomach 12. Just below the clavicle is Stomach 13.

Start by feeling for and massaging St 12, above the clavicle. Go down into the "pocket" a little behind the clavicle. This is often a very sensitive area and, for most people, filled with tension. Massage it gently.

I find it is most helpful to feel both shoulder areas at once with the tips of my first two or three fingers, palms down. I also use the sides of my thumbs, keeping in mind that the thumbs are powerful. It can be tempting to press too hard on the points, so be especially gentle when using your thumbs.

As with any part of lymphatic massage, the release happens while you are searching for the points and discovering places of tension. Very often, in order to find the point, you will have to release the surface tension in the area. Even if you do find it right away, you will need to loosen the area to increase Qi flow to the point.

Now find the drainage sites themselves. They will be felt as lumps of tissue, about the size of the end of your thumb, behind the clavicle bones. They can be felt as small rises within the "pocket" area behind the clavicle bones. They are usually sensitive and give a kind of electric feedback to your hands. As you massage the area, move toward the clavicle bones, because that is where the openings of the ducts are located. Move slowly and gently, with the intention of relaxing and releasing the ducts.

As you do the work, imagine that you are peeling layers of tension and debris from the area, and then moving downward into the "drain" behind the clavicle. You will sometimes feel it release as you reach the end of your sweep, as though it dropped off of the edge. The total distance you are moving at this point is a quarter of an inch or less.

If, after twenty or thirty seconds, you do not feel a slow release, you may be pressing too hard. Start with lighter pressure and sweep gently and slowly. It's also possible that the sensation is too subtle for you to recognize at this point, especially if the person is very tight in this area. Spend a few minutes on this area, but don't overdo it. I often return to the area after I have worked other parts of the body.

The next point is St 13, directly below the clavicle from St 12. Massage the general area on both sides with your fingers and slowly circle inward until you are just massaging the point directly under the clavicle. Apply pressure evenly and then slowly upward, the same pattern as was used with St 12, compressing the lymph and then sweeping it toward the drain. Again, don't try to do too much at once.

After you have a fair amount of release, you may feel a softening of the area, accompanied by the point itself getting smaller and more defined. You will often find this is the case with acupressure points as they release. Don't overwork the area.

RELEASING THE JUGULAR LYMPHATIC TRUNK

As you work on the neck area, be sure that you do not apply any pressure to the trachea (windpipe). Also, work and release only one side of the neck at a time.

Begin releasing the jugular lymphatic trunk by turning the person's head to one side. In your mind, draw an imaginary line down the center of the side of the neck facing you, from the earlobe to the drainage site. This is the approximate location of the jugular lymphatic duct.

This line will pass across the sternocleidomastoid muscle, the large muscle going from the inside tip of the clavicle to the mastoid bone just behind the ear, crossing it about halfway up the neck.

Start massaging about one-half inch above St 12, near the place where the neck joins the shoulders. Pull the skin toward the ear, as far as it goes before it is drawn too taut. For most people, the skin can stretch about half an inch to an inch. Apply pressure to the lymph duct and slowly sink in, allowing the area to melt under your fingers. As it melts, you will feel pulled downward by the skin. Allow your hand to slide downward toward the drainage point, while you maintain a constant level of pressure. You want to do this sweep gently and slowly, never forcing things. As you slide, the skin will slack until you pass the point where you first contacted.

The purpose of pulling the skin up is to be able to massage the tissue deeply without causing a "rope burn" on the neck.

Next, move up to a little above the highest point of your last sweep and do another sweep, again pulling the skin up and sweeping downward. There should be a small amount of overlap between sweeps to ensure that the lymph is carried into the following area.

You may find an area or two that feels hard and immovable. If so, it is important to release the tension in the area or the lymph drainage will be compromised. Do a general neck release, as we covered in chapter 20. After releasing the neck, the lymphatic duct should release more easily.

It will probably take you four to six sweeps before you reach the area just below the ear. Between the jawbone and the mastoid process (the bottom of the bone area that swells just behind the ear, where the sternocleidomastoid muscle attaches) is the styloid process. This thin tube of bone is an attachment point for several muscles. It is a sensitive area, so be very gentle.

In this area, there are the cervical nodes. In the advanced ALR to be covered immediately below, we will release these thoroughly, but for now, gently massage this area. Go into the muscles on the jaw and in front of the ear, then back behind the ear and back at the base of the skull. Gently massage the area under the jaw, starting in the back. Then gently knead the area of the jugular lymphatic duct for ten seconds or so, starting at the bottom by the release point and moving up a little at a time in small downward strokes. This will stimulate the lymph flow and ensure an even release.

ADVANCED RELEASE PATTERNS

These release patterns should be used only after one or two basic release sessions have been completed.

ADVANCED JUGULAR RELEASE

When you got to the area under the earlobe, you may have noticed a hard area that felt like a swollen lymph gland; most people have this to a greater or lesser degree. It is also common for one side to be larger and tighter than the other. Go to just below the area and pull the skin up toward the ear so that the very tips of your thumbs or fingers are on the very bottom of the swollen area, barely on the edge of it, and, again with the very tips of your thumbs or fingers, apply light pressure very slowly in and then downward in the direction of the proper flow. This will often take twenty to thirty seconds to release, sometimes more. Imagine that there is a little plug there that you are dissolving and pushing downward.

Go back and repeat this once or twice for a shorter time and then follow through by sweeping down the jugular duct as far as the skin will comfortably travel. Gently massage the lymph fluid down the length of the jugular duct, then go back, and with the flat of your thumb or finger, pull the skin up a bit and apply gentle pressure directly onto the swollen area, waiting for it to release. As it releases, follow it downward a little. Repeat.

If the release seems very slow or sluggish, roll onto the tips of your fingers and apply gentle pressure to the "plug" until you feel it release, then go back to the body of the swelling. If there is a release, it will feel as though the swelling deflates. The swelling often returns somewhat in a few minutes, which is fine.

Occasionally, there will be little or no release the first time. In this case, *don't press harder.* If you have spent several minutes trying to get the area to release, you can try a hot compress on the area; just a hot washcloth is fine. This can sometimes help the release.

ADVANCED MASTOID RELEASE

Place the heel, or base, of your hands on the mastoid area, the swelling of bone behind the ear. This is most gracefully done by holding the hands palms down and putting the base of the thumbs behind the client's ears, then pivoting the hands so that the heel of each hand is resting on the mastoid while the palm and fingers hold the back of the head. It is helpful to partially lock your fingers behind the client's head and upper neck.

Ask the client to take three slow, deep breaths. As the client inhales, apply firm (but not excessive or painful) pressure to both mastoids, squeezing them between your hands. As the client exhales, release pressure.

What you are doing is pumping the lymph drainage in this area, using the pressure created in the head by the inhalation to press from the inside as you press from the outside.

Next, go back to the swelling below the earlobe and reapply gentle pressure, allowing it to release. You will often notice a difference in the area, either a little thick plug that dissipates as you work on it or a feeling of less thickness and more thin fluid, or both. Sweep down the jugular duct in the same way you came up it, pulling the skin up and sweeping downward several times down toward the drainage point.

ADVANCED SUBMAXILLARY RELEASE

Next, place your fingers in a row under the jaw with the pinky fingers by the back corner of the jaw and the index fingers about an inch from the chin. With your pinky fingers, pull the skin forward and press upward into the submaxillary gland area inside the jaw; allow it to release slowly. As with other areas, slide the fingers back in the direction of flow as far as the skin will allow. Repeat this same procedure with the ring fingers, pulling the skin forward, pressing up superiorly behind the mandible, and sliding the finger back to promote the flow of lymph. Then repeat this same process with the middle and index fingers.

Now move the fingers forward so that the index fingers are under the front of the chin and repeat the whole process starting with the pinky finger. After you are done, sweep the entire area from the chin to the back of the jaw and then down the jugular duct, pulling the skin forward and sweeping as far as the skin will comfortably allow.

RELEASING THE SUBCLAVIAN TRUNK

Next, we will bring our attention to the area just below the clavicle, going out to the armpit. This is the subclavian trunk (there's one on each side), which drains the axillary nodes of the armpit and outer chest. Start by massaging the area of St 13 again. Then draw an imaginary line from St 13 to the armpit; this is the approximate location of the subclavian duct.

In the same way as with the jugular duct, start about one-half inch away from the drainage point and pull the skin taut, toward the armpit. Apply pressure and allow the area to sink in, then sweep inward toward the drainage point. This area is much less sensitive than the neck, but even so, do not use excessive pressure. You want the duct to compress and release in its own time.

Move out to the area a little past the farthest you got out on your last sweep and sweep inward. Again, you want to have some overlapping with your last sweep. Repeat this sweep inward and move outward until you have reached the edge of the armpit.

Feel the very outside of the pectoral muscle on the outside of the chest just below where it connects with the arm. You will be on the corner where the front and the side of the chest meet. If you find any tension or any knots there, massage them out, as they tend to block drainage from the axillary nodes of the armpit as well as the drainage from the lateral aspect of the breast in women.

Finish by massaging inward along the subclavian duct to the drainage point, pressing more firmly to move the ribs slightly. End by pumping the clavicle again.

RELEASING THE INTERCOSTAL TRUNKS

You may want to be beside the client for this part. Start again at St 13, the drainage point below the clavicle. Move about one-half inch in toward the sternum from St 13, pulling the skin toward the sternum as far as it wants to go, then sweep back to the drainage point. This distance can probably be done in one sweep.

Next we will release the intercostal spaces, the spaces between the ribs just adjacent to the sternum. For each space, start by massaging the space to soften it up, then put your finger about a half-inch from the sternum in the space and pull the skin outward, away from the sternum, as far as it wants to go. Sweep inward, and then upward superiorly a little bit as you reach the edge of the sternum. Move down to each intercostal space until you are just past the sternum, where the spaces will begin to be farther out. Five or six intercostal spaces should have been released.

Lastly, place the palm of your hand on the upper sternum and apply gentle pressure as the client breathes out. Repeat this several times, each time moving downward toward the lower sternum.

ADVANCED INTERCOSTAL RELEASE

This advanced treatment pattern should be used only after one or two basic release sessions have been completed.

After you have released the intercostal spaces, do the following technique instead of pumping the sternum. (We call this the "washing machine" release.)

Place the hand that is closer to the client's head just above the clavicle in the area of St 12. Grasp the clavicle, putting your fingers above and as far behind it as you can without causing discomfort; place the heel of your hand on the lower front of the clavicle so that you have a firm grasp on the clavicle.

Place your other hand just below the ribs about halfway down from the sternum to the waist. Grasp the lowest ribs in this area with your fingers behind the ribs as far as you can without discomfort and place the heel of your hand on the front of the ribs, again to get a firm grasp.

Hold on to these areas firmly. Starting slowly and gently to allow the client to get used to it, begin to move your hands in opposite directions. The upper hand moves medially as the lower hand moves laterally and slides down under the ribs; then the upper hand moves outward as the lower moves inward and slides up the ribs. This should cause a gentle twisting of the ribs to squeeze the lymph glands and ducts throughout the ribs while your hands massage the lymphatic drainage point at St 12 and the lymph glands under the lower ribs. It is a bit like patting your head and rubbing your stomach the first few times you do it, but once you get used to it the technique is simple.

Some people are very sensitive in these areas. If you cannot grasp under the ribs or behind the clavicle, do the best you can and rely more on the pressure from the heel of your hands. It is often helpful to have the client place his or her hands on top of yours.

Switch sides and repeat the technique. After this, pump the sternum lightly, starting higher up and moving downward.

RELEASING THE LOWER LYMPHATIC DUCTS

For now, you will do a short massage of the lower thoracic duct and cisterna chyli. Start about two inches below the sternum with the same release pattern you were using with each previous area, this time pulling the skin downward, applying pressure from the flat of several fingers and wait to sink in, then slowly sweep upward to just below the sternum. Move down the centerline, each time about an inch farther so that there is some overlap, until you reach just above the navel.

At this point, take your thumbs and slide them upward with a circular massage from just above the navel to below the sternum. On the bottom of the sternum is the xiphoid process, a sharp point of bone like a little tail on the sternum; this is a sensitive area, so don't press up into the sternum.

ADVANCED LOWER TRUNK RELEASE

This advanced release is used after one or two basic sessions have been completed.

Next, continue this release but move diagonally down and out toward a point halfway between the corner of the pubic bone and the anterior superior iliac spine (ASIS), the bony prominence on the front outside of the upper hips, just below the belt line.

At this point, you will release the inguinal lymph nodes. Using either the heel of your hand or the tips of your four fingers, massage from just inside the ASIS diagonally down and in toward the corner of the pubic bone. Then move back out and down so that you are below the ASIS, about even in height with the pubic bone, and again massage in toward the corner of the pubic bone. Move out and down again to below the height of the pubic bone and massage diagonally up and in to the corner of the pubic bone.

Lastly, sweep diagonally back up to the navel and continue up to just below the sternum.

Repeat this same procedure on the other side, moving diagonally down from the navel area while sweeping upward, then massaging the inguinal lymph nodes. End by sweeping up to the navel and then to below the sternum.

FINISHING UP

End with a massage of the small of the back to stimulate the kidneys. Ask the client to drink a lot of water over the next few days and rest as much as possible. It is also helpful to do some gentle stretching to promote lymphatic flow.

BASIC LYMPHATIC RELEASE
TREATMENT PATTERN

This release should be used during the first one or two sessions. Remember to follow the protocol:

1. Contact skin.
2. Pull skin away from direction of drainage as far as is comfortable.
3. Apply pressure and allow fingers to sink into the tissue.
4. Sweep: slide in direction of drainage; slide skin as far as comfortable.
5. If drainage is poor, release tension in area, then repeat steps 1 through 4.

ALWAYS move the lymph toward the drainage site (St 12 and 13). Release the drainage site, then release farther away from the site, sweeping lymph fluid toward the drainage site. (As when combing long hair, you start at the bottom and comb downward while moving progressively upward.)

1. Massage the small of the back (kidney area) with the client lying on his or her stomach. Sitting above the client's head, rock him or her gently by pushing on the shoulders toward the feet until the whole body rocks. Release St 12 and St 13 on both sides.
2. Starting at St 12, move up the jugular trunk as you are pushing downward. Move toward the earlobe. Release bands of tension only on the sides on which they appear.
3. Massage the jaw muscles, behind the ear, and under the jaw.
4. Release the subclavian trunk, between St 13 and the armpit.
5. Massage from St 13 to the outside of the sternum. Release the broncho-mediastinal trunk by moving down the intercostal spaces, pressing in-

ward and then up. Pump the sternum gently, starting from the top and moving down.

6. Release the thoracic duct and cisterna chyli by starting below the sternum, just below the xiphoid process, and moving downward to just above the navel. Massage upward to below the xiphoid process.

7. Massage the small of the back to stimulate the kidneys.

ADVANCED LYMPHATIC RELEASE
TREATMENT PATTERN

This release should be used only after one or two basic release sessions. Remember to follow the protocol.

1. Contact skin.
2. Pull skin away from direction of drainage as far as comfortable.
3. Apply pressure and allow fingers to sink into the tissue.
4. Sweep: slide in direction of drainage; slide skin as far as comfortable.
5. If drainage is poor, release tension in area, then repeat steps 1 through 4.

ALWAYS move the lymph toward the drainage site (St 12 and 13). Release the drainage site, then release farther away from the site, sweeping lymph fluid toward the drainage site. (As when combing long hair, you start at the bottom and comb downward while moving progressively upward.)

1. Massage the small of the back (kidney area) with the client lying on his or her stomach. Sitting above the client's head, rock him or her gently by pushing on the shoulders toward the feet until the whole body rocks. Release St 12 and St 13 on both sides.

2. Starting at St 12, move up the jugular trunk as you are pushing downward. Move toward the earlobe. Release bands of tension only on the sides on which they appear.

3. Release the cervical lymph nodes just below the ears, starting on the very lower edge. Sweep down the jugular trunk.

4. Compress the mastoid bone on both sides while the client is breathing in; repeat three times. Sweep down the jugular trunk, taking care to clear the upper part of the trunk.

5. Release the submandibular nodes under the jaw, sweeping back with each of the fingers and then repeating with the fingers closer to the chin. Sweep the jugular trunk again.

6. Release the subclavian trunk, between St 13 and the armpit. Massage

the axillary nodes in the armpit area. Release any blockage at the edge of pectoral by the armpit. Sweep back to St 13.

7. Massage inward from St 13 to the outside of the sternum. Release the bronchomediastinal trunk by moving down the intercostal spaces, sweeping inward and then up.

8. Perform the "washing machine" release. Pump the sternum gently, starting from the top and moving lower.

9. Release the lower thoracic duct and cisterna chyli by starting below the sternum, just below the xiphoid process, and moving downward to just above the navel. Sweep upward to below the xiphoid process.

10. Release the lumbar trunks and massage the inguinal nodes inward toward the corner of the pubic bone three times: diagonally down, directly inward, and diagonally up.

11. Sweep up the lumbar trunks to the navel and the thoracic duct to just below the sternum.

12. Pump the sternum, moving upward. Massage the small of the back to stimulate the kidneys.

Acupressure lymphatic release is one of the most important parts of an acupressure treatment because its healing effects are so essential in today's environment. Each of us encounters many environmental toxins in our food, water, and air. All of them have the potential to tax our blood-cleansing organs beyond their limits and eventually accumulate in our interstitial fluid, where they can cause real problems for our health. Acupressure lymphatic release addresses all of these concerns. It opens the system, promotes movement and release of both old and new poisons, and helps to strengthen our immune systems against any future threat.

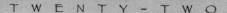

Exercises for a Full Body Treatment

You can give yourself a full body treatment every day simply by doing the following ancient Daoist exercises, each of which was designed to individually open and clear a specific meridian. Since the Chinese also saw the intimate and inextricable relationship between the mind and body, each exercise is also designed to expand your understanding of yourself and the world around you. If practiced daily, the exercises will promote purification of the blood and bodily systems, improve breathing and posture, strengthen your vital center—or the source of your energy—release tension, dramatically improve your health, and help transform your view of yourself and life in general.

As you do these exercises, concentrate deeply on the movements and the breathing. Use your imagination to feel the energy flowing through you as it is stimulated by the exercise. Keep your eyes half-closed, your tongue resting lightly on the roof of your mouth, and your muscles relaxed. With each movement, try to get a sense of what the Daoists called "thick air," the feeling that you are pushing through molasses. Slow and steady movement will energize you and bring a feeling of strength and resiliency.

HORSE STANCE:
KIDNEY MERIDIAN

Many of the Daoist exercises, as well as other martial arts, incorporate the horse stance. It is said to magnify the power of any exercise and to be very beneficial when done with meditative breathing techniques.

Stand with the feet apart, shoulder-width or more, with the knees bent and the thighs spread so that the knees are over the toes, shinbones vertical, as if you were riding a horse. When holding this position for very long, such as in meditation, the knees may begin to shake.

LOOSENING SINEWS:
SOURCE POINTS OF ALL ORGAN MERIDIANS

The extremities of the body are very important from an acupressure point of view. It is there that the meridian energy changes from yin to yang and vice versa, and it is these areas where some of the most important acupoints are found. By relieving tension in the wrists and ankles, one helps to promote the free circulation of energy in the meridians.

While standing on one foot, roll the ankle of the other foot several times in both directions. Shake the leg until the foot shakes freely. Repeat this with the other foot, then shake the arms so the hands shake freely. Briefly massage the wrists.

BENDING:
KIDNEY AND LARGE INTESTINE ORGANS; GALL BLADDER
AND BLADDER MERIDIANS

These are variations on the "life prolonging" exercises of Daoist Qi Gong. They stimulate the kidneys and large intestines, relieve tension in the back and shoulders, and stimulate the bladder and gall bladder meridians. The life prolonging exercises build Qi storage, thought to be in the kidneys, which is essential to longevity and good health.

With the feet planted shoulder-width apart, lock the fingers together with the palms down. Bend down with the knees straight or slightly bent and stretch your arms down. Sway from side to side, moving from the hips and waist. Breathe in and straighten up, allow the arms to take a diving position over the head, and bend back, arching the neck and back. Breathe out. Stand up straight and lock your fingers together behind your lower back. The palms should face the floor. Bend forward and raise your arms upward, so that the palms face the ceiling.

Return to standing with feet spread and release your locked fingers. Bend to one side while facing front, letting one arm slide down the outside of the thigh while the other arm raises over your head in an arc to the side; breathe in. Return to an upright position while exhaling and repeat on the other side. Do this a few times on both sides.

BACK TWIST:
ALL ORGANS, ESPECIALLY KIDNEYS

Massages the internal organs and the lymph system, relieves blockages in the back, hips, and shoulders.

Spread the feet wider than shoulder-width. Twist the torso, slowly at first, while allowing the arms to swing freely and keeping the feet planted. Movement should come from the waist with the back straight. The breath should be held and then slowly exhaled, as this serves to loosen the spine from the bottom up.

NECK ROLL:
NECK MERIDIANS, ESPECIALLY BLADDER, GALL BLADDER, TRIPLE WARMER, AND SMALL INTESTINE

This exercise helps relieve neck and shoulder tension, allows better circulation to the brain, and helps to realign neck vertebrae.

Do this exercise carefully, especially if you have had neck problems in the past. If you feel any pain or constriction, stop the exercise and apply pressure to the muscles on the sides of the vertebrae in that area, then continue. If you feel sharp pain, simply tilt the head to the sides, front, and back instead of doing a circular motion.

With your feet spread and knees slightly bent, roll your head slowly in one direction. Start with the jaw closed, and with each rotation, open the jaw a little further. Repeat this in the opposite direction. Shake the head several times slowly, increasing speed to a moderate rate. If there is any pain like headache, slow down until the pain is gone or barely noticeable.

OPENING THE BOW:
LUNG AND LARGE INTESTINE MERIDIANS

This exercise especially stimulates the large intestine and lung meridians, two of the most important meridians for the expulsion of toxins from the body. This exercise is good for cleansing the body of wastes, cleansing the blood, and promoting good oxygenation, thus making it an excellent brain exercise.

In the horse stance, form a claw with the right hand while pointing the left index finger straight up with the tips of the thumb and the middle fingers touching. You will bring the arms up as if shooting a very large bow to your left, the right arm drawing the string and the left finger signifying the bow. Keep the right (claw) elbow down and start the hand near the chin. Push out with the left hand to the side, breathing out, and at the same time draw back the right hand. The left index finger should point straight up. Bring the arms back to the chest, palms facing each other, and repeat on the other side. Keep switching and repeating several times.

RAISE HANDS SEPARATELY:
LUNG, LARGE INTESTINE, CIRCULATION/PERICARDIUM, TRIPLE WARMER, HEART, AND SMALL INTESTINE

In addition to massaging the meridians of the arm (Lu, LI, C/P, TW, Ht, SI) and helping to relax the shoulders, this exercise helps to change your movement pattern, helping you to move in the most tension-free manner possible. Most people exert far more energy than is needed for a given task.

In the Horse Stance, have your arms to the sides with elbows back, wrists by the waist, hands palm-up in fists, and breathe in. Exhale as you slowly punch out with one arm, rotating the forearm so that the palm is down when the arm is extended. Retract the arm to its original position while breathing in. Repeat with the other arm. Return to the original position and, while breathing out, bring the first arm to your side by tracing a downward arc with the fist. The forearm will rotate so the palm faces down. As you bring the arm back to your side, extend it directly out, away from the body. Slowly bring the arm down and then return the arm to its original position, retracing the arc and breathing in. Repeat with the other arm. Start at the beginning and repeat this exercise several times, trying to use as little effort as possible so the arms seem to float.

SQUEEZE KNEE:
STOMACH, SPLEEN, KIDNEY, BLADDER, LIVER, AND GALL BLADDER MERIDIANS

This is a stretch for the leg meridians (Ki, Bl, Lv, GB, Sp, St), especially the stomach meridian. It also strengthens the knees and ankles and improves balance.

With feet spread wide and hands in diving position, fingers locked, lower yourself down on one leg with the other leg straight, its foot turned outward forty-five degrees. Go down as far as comfortable, pointing the toes. Keep the back fairly straight, hips facing forward. Do this on both sides several times, then do it with both feet pointing straight ahead.

Two Hands Push Sky:
General Qi Flow and Energy Building

This exercise helps calm and center one, promoting good balance while helping to unblock all the meridians.

From a normal standing position, raise the arms to the sides, palms out, and lock the fingers over the head, palms facing down. This is done while breathing in. Rotate the forearms so the palms face up, fingers still loosely locked, and push upward while raising the body up from the toes and then lowering your body, breathing out. Lower the arms to your sides with palms facing out, wrists bent, and continue the arc up to the abdomen as if lifting the air in front, breathing in. Rotate the hands and push down toward the floor, breathing out. Do this several times.

Shake Head and Wave Tail:
Kidney and Large Intestine Organs; Waist Meridians

This exercise is for the lower back and kidneys. It also aids in balancing the muscle tone of the torso.

In the Horse Stance, place the hands on the upper thighs in front. Take a breath and bend down to one side while keeping the legs bent and moving from the waist in an arc. Breathe out as you reach the bottom of the arc (your head is down and in front of you) and swing up the other side. Repeat several times, then go in the opposite direction several times as well.

Energy Exercises:
Building the Qi

This exercise can be done concurrently with the next two: After you finish the Energy Pump, move right into Centering; repeat this seven to nine times. Afterwards, return to the Energy Pump, this time moving into Focused Energy; repeat seven to nine times. End with one last cycle of the Energy Pump.

The Energy Pump

This exercise focuses your concentration, dispels distracting thoughts, and builds the Qi of the kidneys.

In the Horse Stance, place the hands in front of the abdomen with palms up, fingers loosely locked. Bring the hands up to low chest level while breathing in and almost straightening the knees. Rotate the forearms so that the palms are facing down and lower the arms while breathing out and bending into the Horse Stance again. Do this several times until the mind is clear and free of distractions.

CENTERING

This exercise, along with helping to center the mind and body, is for gathering energy into the lower warmer and the kidneys.

While raising the hands in the Energy Pump, continue in an arc over the head and down to the sides; allow the fingers to unlock and bend the wrists so the palms face out, straightening the arms. Breathe in while raising, out while lowering. Return the hands to the original position and repeat seven to nine times or until your mind feels centered and refreshed.

FOCUSED ENERGY

This exercise is good for tension, low energy, and anxiety. Relieves Qi blockages, especially in the chest and abdomen (the Great Central Channel).

In the Horse Stance, raise the hands with palms facing up, as in Two Hands Push Sky, while almost straightening the legs and breathing in. Cross the wrists, palms facing to the opposite sides, the sides of the wrists touching. Bring them down the front while bending the knees, and breathe out. Continue the arc out and up again into the same exercise, crossing wrists on the opposite sides of the hands. Repeat seven to nine times or until you feel very grounded.

As you sweep downward, end by slowing as your hands move down toward the floor and hold them there for a moment while you bring your awareness back to your surroundings.

If done regularly, these exercises can have a powerful effect on every aspect of your life. Your overall energy and vitality will be boosted enormously. There will be significant effects on your consciousness. You will become acutely aware of your body and its subtle and obvious powers. Your intuition will grow stronger, and your capacity to concentrate will improve dramatically. In short, these exercises can change your life.

The Acupressure Facial

Beauty is the word we use to describe a condition in which many small, individual characteristics are joined in harmony and balance. Such qualities that we refer to as good, true, full of radiant energy, and even love are all implicit in that which is beautiful.

When I confront something that is beautiful, I am instantly excited, alert, alive. Before coming into the presence of beauty, my life energy, my Qi, was tied up with other matters; I was preoccupied and somehow duller. But once I stand before that which is beautiful, I am awakened to all that upholds, sustains, and enriches life. I am more alive. Life and death are constantly struggling within each of us, and the single indication that life is winning is the beauty that surrounds us and radiates from within us. Beauty and life are one, just as ugliness is a harbinger of onrushing death. Consequently, whenever we encounter beauty, something inside of us leaps with joy, because all of us seek the beauty of life.

Therefore it is natural that all of us would pursue beauty, especially our own beauty, just as it is natural to pursue our own truth. We might say that beauty is simply the artistic—or harmonious—presentation of truth. Beauty and truth are inextricably joined, because both fundamentally support life. That is why the face of an old man or woman that radiates energy, honesty, goodness, and truth is beautiful. When you confront such a face, your own inner truth feels nurtured, enriched, and even magnified. For something to be truly beautiful, it must be founded on what is true. That's why the face of an older person who possesses the characteristics just mentioned transcends all cultural stereotypes of the latest fad-definition of beauty.

Conversely, something inside of us rebels whenever we are confronted with a face that is covered with too much makeup. There is something dishonest in all that paint and clay.

The Chinese recognized that life is an entity, a substance, that permeates the body and radiates from it. Life force, or Qi, is the foundation of beauty. Those who live in harmony with the laws of life are imbued with Qi. They glow with it. This is why artists depict saints with halos, and why artistic renderings of Jesus and the Buddha show them literally glowing with life energy.

All of us have it within our power to boost the life energy within us by using acupressure and by living in harmony with our own underlying truths. Acupressure can be used to boost and enhance the life force flowing throughout the body, and specifically in the face. Qi is the basis for all healing and restoration. The absence of Qi is the basis for aging, sagging tissues, and wrinkled skin.

When Qi is diminished, we experience the signs of aging throughout the body. Diminished Qi is reflected most notably in the face in the following ways:

- The skin loses its elasticity. It sags more and is prone to wrinkle.

- Tissues below the surface congest and adhere to the skin. This results from long-term muscular tension, and facial injuries, and it leads to wrinkles.

- Facial markings, from weak internal organs, appear; especially from chronic stress within the nervous system. These may be creases, wrinkles, and sagging tissue.

- Skin takes on an unhealthy appearance and tone, the result of poor digestion, assimilation, and elimination, as well as poor circulation of blood, lymph, and Qi throughout the body.

The regular application of an acupressure facial can restore Qi and youthful vitality and radiance to the face, just as regular acupressure can restore Qi and healing throughout the body.

Chinese medicine sees the face as an indicator of our internal health—

weak kidneys show up as dark circles under our eyes, for example. A Chinese doctor might say that the best facial treatment is to keep the whole body healthy. He would also recommend a regular routine of treating the face with acupressure. In addition to stimulating Qi flow in the body, a regular acupressure facial treatment will help to keep the face flexible and youthful. The treatment reduces facial muscle tension—which in time can engrave lines on your face—and increases blood and lymph circulation. It brings essential oxygen to skin cells and carries away cellular waste products, as well as stimulates key acupressure points.

NECK AND SHOULDER RELEASE

We begin the acupressure facial by relaxing the neck and shoulders. Tension in the neck and shoulders reduces circulation to the face, and uneven tension in the neck increases muscular tension in the face. Similarly, nerve inflammation in the neck will irritate the nerves going to the face. I start every acupressure facial with a neck and shoulder release.

Start by massaging the shoulders and neck. As you massage, move and stretch the neck and shoulders to increase the release of tension. Release the points of the shoulder release pattern—Small Intestine 9 and 10 above the back of the armpit, Triple Warmer 15 at the top inside corner of the shoulder blade, Gall Bladder 21 on top of the shoulders at the base of the neck, and Gall Bladder 20 under the back of the head.

Next, massage the head to increase circulation and to relax the muscles. Most of us carry a great deal of tension in the head muscles; try to relax these muscles by massaging and stretching them. A great technique is to slide the scalp, pulling it together and stretching it apart, first to the sides, and then to the front and back.

The remainder of the treatment can be done with or without lotion or oil. If you aren't using lotion or oil, make sure you don't overstretch the skin, as this can damage it and actually do more harm than good.

You may treat yourself or a partner to the acupressure facial. If you're working on yourself, try to stay as relaxed as possible—lying down, if you wish. If you're working on someone else, have the person lie on his or her back while you sit in front of the person's head. (This is the same position we use for the neck and shoulder release.)

STIMULATING THE LYMPH SYSTEM

The lymph system is one of the least understood functions of the body, and yet it performs the vital function of removing toxic waste products from the cells. The face has an intricate network of lymph vessels. A regular acupressure facial will stimulate the lymphatic drainage of the head. This is also an excellent sinus drainage protocol.

Start at the base of the neck, three fingers out from the inner point of the collarbone (clavicle). Just above the clavicle is Stomach 12, at the bottom of the jugular lymphatic trunk, which drains the head. Massage this area with the tips of your fingers using very gentle circular strokes, and as you massage begin moving straight up the neck to a point just behind the jaw, slightly behind and above SI 17—this is the path of the jugular lymph duct. We will call this the jaw point.

From the jaw point, massage forward onto the jaw. You want to massage the face such that everything moves toward this jaw point. With the lymph, you want to always be massaging in the direction of drainage. As when you comb your hair, if you try to start from the top it will get tangled. If you start from the bottom, combing downward, and then each time move up a little closer to the top, you can easily work through all the knots.

As you massage the face, imagine that you are moving the lymph back toward the jaw point and downward. Using circular motions of the fingertips, massage in front of the ear all the way to the sides of the forehead. Massage forward a little toward the nose and then massage back down to the jaw point.

Massage from this point back to the forehead, then across the top of the forehead, and down to just above the eyebrows. Continue massaging with the fingertips under the eyebrows (above the eyes). Now put your fingers just below the eyes at the sides of the nose and massage up onto the bridge of the nose and around the top of the eyes, then back down to the sides of the eyes. Next, massage down to the jaw. Start again at the sides of the nose and massage under the eyes, then down to the jaw. Start a third time at the sides of the nose a little farther down, and massage back to the jaw point. Next, massage from the upper lip back to the jaw point, then just below the mouth to the jaw point, then last, massage from the front of the chin back to the jaw point.

Now massage the lymph nodes under the jaw. If you are working on someone else, place the tips of your fingers under the jaw at a point about halfway between the back of the jaw and the chin. If you're working on yourself, use the flat of your thumb in the same spot. Use gentle circular massage, then start again just behind the chin and massage all the way back.

RELEASING MUSCLE TENSION

Next, we will release muscular tension. Probably the tightest muscles in the face are in the jaw. The two main muscles are the masseter, which stretches between the bottom of the jaw and the cheekbones, and the temporalis, which stretches from the bottom of the jaw under the cheekbone to the front of the ear and up above the temple. Start by massaging these muscles and stretching them. Have the person open his or her jaw wide and relax it while you massage both with and across the fibers of the muscles. Resist the temptation to press really hard; these muscles, especially the masseter, can be very unyielding. You may be tempted to use excess force to release the tension but it won't help.

One point that can be very helpful is St 6, which you can find by starting at the back corner of the jaw and moving one finger up and one finger forward. The point will often be a little knot and will be sore to the touch. Release this point and the masseter and temporalis will relax over the next several hours. Also, feel for any tension or soreness in the temple area and back toward the scalp and ears and release these points.

There are also muscles in the forehead. These muscles tend to get tight with stress, digestive problems, or liver irritation. The muscles are not obvious; feel on the forehead for underlying creases. These creases are like the furrows after a field is plowed. You want to "push the dirt" back into the furrow. You will notice when you feel the crease that the muscles feel like they have separated and pulled back from the crease. Find the full area outside the crease and push it back into the crease.

Once you have done this, use a dispersive circular massage to clear any congestion and to move the lymph back down toward the drainage, feeling for deep muscular tension or adhesions. Make sure you release between the eyebrows especially; these creases, which correspond to liver and spleen problems, are vertical rather than the horizontal lines on the rest of the forehead.

Now go across the forehead again, but this time apply pressure and release with your fingertips. Start at the top of the forehead and work in a grid pattern, pressing each point for two to three seconds, across and then back a little lower until you have released down to the eyebrows. The pressure should be firm but not painful; again, you are waiting for the area to release without brute force. Wait until the muscles melt under your fingers.

Next, release the orbits of the eyes using this same direct pressure with your fingertips, starting on the inside and up above the eyes, then back down under. Finish with a dispersive circular massage around the eyes, out from the nose above the eyes and back toward the nose underneath.

Now, move down to the cheeks. Massage through the entire area, feeling for deep muscular tension or adhesion—places where the skin doesn't slide across the muscles. Feel especially under the cheekbones. Now go through the entire area again, but this time apply direct pressure with your fingertips in a grid pattern, starting below the eyes and moving in a crisscross pattern until you reach the upper gums. Finish with a dispersive circular massage of the area, moving back toward the ear and down to the jaw point.

Next, massage through the jaw area, starting from the chin and moving back, using the gentle circular massage strokes. Release the jaw area using direct pressure with your fingertips starting at the base of the teeth and moving back, then moving forward a little lower, then back again a little lower until you have released the entire area. End by using a dispersive circular massage of the area.

A GENTLE WRAP-UP

Massage the entire face using the flat of your fingers with a very gentle circular motion, starting at the centerline and moving back to the point on the jaw. Massage the scalp using your fingertips, starting from the top and moving down to the neck. Now massage the neck downward again, using your whole hands with a kneading motion. Massage the shoulders, then end by massaging the feet to draw excess energy away from the head.

Using this acupressure facial once or twice a week can make a tremendous difference over a month or two. Remember that you want to err on the side of being gentle, especially when working on yourself. We tend to be a lot harder on ourselves than on others because we want to change our condition fast.

FIVE DAILY ACUPRESSURE ACTIVITIES TO ENHANCE YOUR BEAUTY

Here is a short series of acupressure points to stimulate every day, preferably before bed or first thing in the morning, to enhance and magnify your beauty.

When stimulating each point, use gentle but firm pressure and a very slight circular motion over each point, for about five seconds. Start by briskly rubbing your hands together to get the Qi moving in your hands and fingers.

1. Gently, but firmly, press the points around the orbit of each eye, starting at the inside and moving out over the eye, then back under, pressing a total of eight points. If you were looking at another person's right eye as a clock, you would start at 3:00, then go to counterclockwise to 1:30, 12:00, 10:30, etc. when you are done, massage around the eyes with very gentle pressure in this same direction, just enough to move the Qi and relax

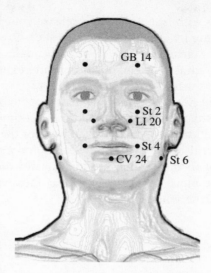

ACUPRESSURE FACE LIFT POINTS

the eyes (you can use an eye cream). End by placing the heels of your palms over the eyes for five to ten seconds.

2. Press the following points: GB 14 (in the center of the forehead directly above the eyes), St 2 (one finger below the center lower orbit of each eye), LI 20 (outside the nostrils), St 4 (at the corners of the mouth), CV 24 (in the center of the crease between the lower lip and the chin), St 6 (by the corner of the jaw in the muscle).

3. Press under the jaw with the sides of your thumbs, starting near the front of the chin and moving back. When you get to the back of the jaw, start behind the ears and massage down the sides and toward the front of the neck with the flat of your fingers.

4. Massage the back of your head, down the back of your neck, and into the shoulders. Use a brisk, Qi-moving approach. Stretch your neck to each side and massage the stretched side down into the shoulders.

5. Do the following exercise to increase oxygen and blood flow to the head: With the feet planted shoulder-width apart, lock your fingers together with the palms down. Bend down with the knees straight or slightly bent and stretch your arms down. Sway from side to side, moving from the hips and waist. Breathe in and straighten up, allow the arms to take a diving position over the head, and bend backward, arching the neck and back. As you breathe out, lower your arms and clasp your hands behind your back. This will make the arms point up when you're leaning forward and point down while you're arching back.

Return to standing with feet spread and release your locked fingers. Bend to one side while facing front, letting one arm slide down the outside of the thigh while the other arm raises over your head in an arc to the side, breathing in. Return to an upright position while exhaling and repeat on the other side. Do this a few times on both sides.

In a week, you will notice an improvement in your skin tone and in the fitness of the muscles that support your skin. If continued over a month or two you will see significant improvement in both of these areas. Gradually, your underlying natural beauty will be revealed and enhanced, all because you boosted Qi flow to the points, meridians, and muscles of your face. Not only will you be more beautiful, but your face will be radiant and a clearer image of the true you.

Foot Reflexology

Reflexology is a natural health care treatment more than four thousand years old. Cave drawings depicting the practice—dated as long ago as 2330 B.C.—have been found in Egypt. Reflexology was also utilized by the ancient Chinese and Japanese.

Foot reflexology is one of the simplest, yet most powerful techniques you can learn. Reflexology, as it's known today, is based on the theory that the feet have "reflex zones" that correspond to the body's organs and systems. These zones or points are massaged to relieve stress, promote healing, and restore balance to meridians that are blocked. Practitioners believe that nerve pathways in the feet connect these "reflex zones" to every organ and system in the body. By stimulating the reflex zones, practitioners send additional Qi through the nerves to specific areas of the body, and thus promote healing.

Reflexology should not be considered a substitute for acupressure, simply because it does not have nearly the same effect. Acupressure is the more effective practice because it works directly on acupressure points, which generate the more powerful charge of Qi along the meridian and to specific organs. As an adjunct practice, however, reflexology can be an important and effective tool.

In the early 1930s, physical therapist Eunice Ingham studied the response of different parts of the body to foot reflexology. She documented numerous cases in which reflexology increased

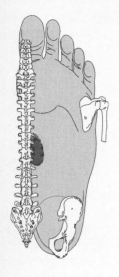
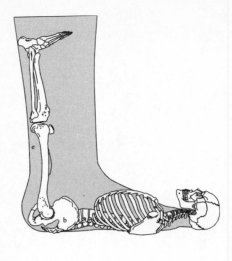

the rate of healing in diseased organs. From her research she devised a map of the feet that mirrors the human body.

The reflexology map I use in Integrative Acupressure is similar to Ingham's, but has been adjusted to reflect the more normal population I work with. What I discovered through treating hundreds of patients, and correlating what I found with other forms of diagnosis, was that many of the reflex zones of the foot became larger when its corresponding organ or structure was irritated. Since most of Ingham's subjects were ill, this caused a distortion of the "map" she created.

The concept behind reflexology is simple: points on the feet reflect the different areas of the body. The left foot reflects the left side of the body; the right foot the right side (i.e., ear points on the right foot correspond to the right ear). The toes reflect the head, the arches and insteps are the waist and low back, and the heels are the pelvis. The spine runs along the inside of the arch where the two feet are closest, from the farthest knuckle of the big toe to just before the heel.

Working on the areas associated with a particular organ or structure, you will find tight or painful spots that indicate excessive energy and some degree of stagnation. By massaging the area, you will boost Qi flow and stimulate the organ or structure that area of the foot represents. You usually need to use deeper pressure with reflexology than with other acupressure methods. There will be some sensitive places but the overall treatment should not be a painful process.

The natural tendency when working on someone else's feet is to face the client from the bottoms of his feet. This is not the best position, however.

It forces you to use your thumbs, when the fingers are actually better suited to most reflexology work. With the person lying on a bed or massage table, sit by his knee and face his feet, reaching around and over the foot to massage the reflexology points with your fingers.

On the accompanying reflexology chart, notice that each zone has a letter in it, referenced by a key below the chart. The reflexology zones we will concentrate on for this complete treatment are the eliminative organs, lymphatic system, endocrine glands and reproductive organs, heart, and digestive system.

In giving a complete reflexology treatment, begin with the eliminative organs. These organs—the kidneys, large intestine, lungs, liver, and gall bladder—cleanse the blood of toxins. To start with any other organs or tissues would increase the amount of toxins in the blood, which would increase stress on the eliminative organs. By stimulating the eliminative organs first, we prepare them for whatever toxins are released when working on other organs or tissues. The treatment will then move to the spleen and and the rest of the lymphatic system, including the endocrine glands, and other major organs.

Start with an overall massage of the right foot with the fingers, briskly getting the blood moving and beginning the process of loosening the muscles.

A. ELIMINATIVE ORGANS

KIDNEYS, BLADDER, AND URETER TUBES

Start to massage the kidney area on the right foot. On the inside bones of the arch you will find a bump halfway between the heel and the tip of the big toe. This is the first cuneiform—and the site of the kidney locator bump. Massage this area deeply. Next, move directly under the arch from here, with your fingers as close as possible to the edge of the arch, and feel for a gristly knot deep in the tissues. This is the kidney and adrenal area; there is a reflexology point for each. One or the other will probably be tight. The adrenal point is half a finger toward the big toe from the kidney locator bump. Just behind that knot is a larger knot, which is the kidney point. Knowing which knot is tight is important: if the adrenal knot is tight, problems with physical or emotional stress are likely; if the kidney point is tighter, excessive stagnation and toxicity within the kidneys is usually the problem.

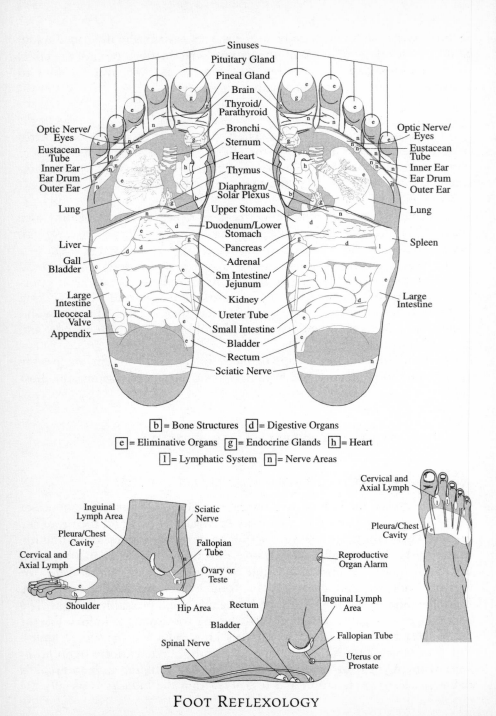

| Sinuses |
| Pituitary Gland |
| Pineal Gland |
| Brain |
| Thyroid/Parathyroid |
| Bronchi |
| Sternum |
| Heart |
| Thymus |
| Diaphragm/Solar Plexus |
| Upper Stomach |
| Duodenum/Lower Stomach |
| Pancreas |
| Adrenal |
| Sm Intestine/Jejunum |
| Kidney |
| Ureter Tube |
| Small Intestine |
| Bladder |
| Rectum |
| Sciatic Nerve |

Optic Nerve/Eyes
Eustacean Tube
Inner Ear
Ear Drum
Outer Ear
Lung
Liver
Gall Bladder
Large Intestine
Ileocecal Valve
Appendix

Optic Nerve/Eyes
Eustacean Tube
Inner Ear
Ear Drum
Outer Ear
Lung
Spleen
Large Intestine

b = Bone Structures   d = Digestive Organs
e = Eliminative Organs   g = Endocrine Glands   h = Heart
l = Lymphatic System   n = Nerve Areas

Inguinal Lymph Area
Pleura/Chest Cavity
Cervical and Axial Lymph
Shoulder
Sciatic Nerve
Fallopian Tube
Ovary or Teste
Hip Area

Cervical and Axial Lymph
Pleura/Chest Cavity

Reproductive Organ Alarm
Inguinal Lymph Area
Fallopian Tube
Uterus or Prostate

Rectum
Bladder
Spinal Nerve

FOOT REFLEXOLOGY

Next, massage down the inside of the arch toward the heel, angling inward so you reach the edge of the arch just before you reach the heel. You will feel a furrow between the muscles that you can follow downward. This is the reflex zone for the ureter tube, the tube that carries urine from the kidneys to the bladder. At the edge of the bottom of the arch, just a finger's distance from the bone of the heel, is a soft, almost hollow area about the size of the tip of your thumb. This is the bladder zone. Massage these areas thoroughly.

Reflexology is a useful tool for diagnosis as well as treatment. For example, many people with recurrent bladder infections will have sensitivity in the ureter tube area. Massaging it and releasing any congestion will help. Of course, the origin of the problem is the kidneys, which are not adequately filtering the urine because of too little fluids, excessive acids, too much stress, or other causes.

LARGE INTESTINE

Next, work your way across the transverse section of the large intestine zone from the kidney area, massaging to the other side of the sole. Feel for any lumps or bumps, which would indicate obstruction or spasm in the colon. Also feel for general fullness, indicating stagnation and putrefaction (fermenting food). When you reach the other side of the foot, work your way down to just short of the heel. If you press deeply, you will feel the edge of the calcaneus (heel bone)—move anteriorly (forward) just to the soft side of this area. This is the appendix and ileocecal valve area, the beginning of the large intestine, known as the cecum. Feel for fullness or knots, then massage it for a bit. If you find specific problem areas, refer to the appropriate chapter for complete treatment of that organ or system.

LUNGS AND SINUSES

Most Westerners do not think of the lungs as eliminative organs, but in fact they eliminate carbon dioxide, which is toxic and acidic, and other toxic gases and fumes formed from chemicals like formaldehyde and pesticides.

The lung zone in reflexology is the pad of the foot under the second through fifth toes. Under the second toe area is the bronchial area. Usually in smokers, this area will feel empty, tight and "dry," though sometimes it will feel full and congested. City dwellers constantly exposed to dirty air often have congestion in the lower lung area as well as irritation in the bronchi.

Massage the bronchial area as well as the top of the foot, in the pleura/

chest cavity area. If the lungs are not cleared adequately by the lymph, the pleural lining around the lungs will be affected. If this area is chronically congested, it can lead to pleurisy.

The sinuses are another mucous membrane that serves an eliminative function. Any toxins not removed through the lymph drainage of the neck and the blood must leave through the sinuses. I often see people with both sinus and neck problems. The tension in the neck blocks lymphatic drainage from the head, so the overflow tries to go out through the sinuses. The sinuses also become overloaded in patients with digestive problems such as dysbiosis and fermentation. (See chapter 27 on dysbiosis and leaky gut syndrome.)

The reflexology areas for the sinuses are the tips of the toes—as small an area as you can pinch and still have a firm grasp of the toe. Massage these with a rolling motion.

Now is a good time to repeat all you have done so far on the opposite foot, beginning with an overall massage on the left foot. You will notice on the chart that the large intestine area on the left foot, unlike the right foot, is C-shaped, with the sigmoid colon traversing just in front of the heel.

LIVER AND GALL BLADDER

Next you will treat the liver, which is represented on the right foot only. The liver zone is located just posterior to the pad of the right foot, behind the fourth and fifth toes. Feel for the edge of the pad where the tougher skin meets the soft skin. You will be able to feel the edge of the ends of the fourth and fifth metatarsal bones. In the soft area posterior to them, the liver and gall bladder areas take up a space about two fingers' distance square.

Imagine the liver area being square, with the gall bladder zone making up the bottom inside of the square. Massage this square area on the foot and feel for congestion, bumps, puffiness, or soreness. The area of the liver closest to the gall bladder on the square is more affected by recent events and tends to clear more quickly—I call it "new liver." The farther away from this area you go, the more it reflects the long-term picture of the liver: past toxic exposures and damage that affected your liver, even into childhood. The outer and upper edges of the liver area tend to be harder and don't release as easily.

After completing the liver area, return to the left foot.

B. LYMPHATIC SYSTEM

SPLEEN

The spleen area is the same as the liver, only on the left foot—and a slightly smaller area. It is only one finger from top to bottom, and less than two fingers wide. If the spleen is irritated, this area will feel like a gristly knot, indicating some chronic immune system activity such as is found with allergies, dysbiosis, toxicity, or chronic illness. Massage this area.

The spleen is also our entrance into the inner body. All the other eliminative organs discharge either into the digestive system or directly to the outside world, but the spleen, along with the rest of the lymphatic system, discharges into the blood. Clear the other eliminative organs before activating the lymphatic system strongly.

LYMPH AREAS

The most important area of the lymphatic system to release is the actual spot where the lymph drains back into the blood. This is located behind the clavicle at the base of the neck (refer to chapter 21, "Acupressure Lymphatic Release"). This spot is reflected in the area of the webbing between the first and second toes. Massage this area thoroughly, all the way up to the top of the space between the first and second metatarsal bones, into the lung/pleura area on the chart. This reflects the bronchomediastinal trunk along the edge of the sternum, which drains the lungs and medial breast area, and the upper thoracic duct, which drains the lower body.

Massage between each of the toes from the webbing up into the foot to release the subclavian trunk, which drains the lymph nodes under the armpit and the lateral breast area.

By the medial and lateral malleoli are the groin lymph areas. Massage the area just under and in front of the lateral malleolus (the outer groin area) and below the medial malleolus in an arc shape (the inner groin area).

Lastly, massage the entire foot, twisting and flexing it as though you were squeezing out a sponge (though not so much as to cause pain; this should feel good). End with a vigorous friction massage.

C. ENDOCRINE GLANDS AND REPRODUCTIVE ORGANS

The pituitary gland area is located in the center of the last section of the big toe. If there are problems with the pituitary gland, you will be able to feel a tight little bead by pressing in deep here.

The thyroid gland point is shown on most charts as very large, covering the section of the ball of the foot behind the big toe. My experience is that it is normally much smaller, located at the top of this same area, pressing into the bone at the base of the first phalange of the big toe. This is also the area for the parathyroid, which is usually not tangible unless it is problematic. If it is problematic, you will be able to feel distinct beads in the thyroid area.

The thymus gland area is under the ball of the first toe, pressing into the edge of the bone (near the tip of the first metatarsal). This is frequently sore, indicating that the immune functioning is compromised.

The pancreas area is under the ball of the foot in the soft area below the second through fourth toes. As you can see from the chart, the area on the right foot is smaller than on the left because of the size of the liver. Even so, the right side is usually more important, corresponding to the head of the pancreas, which contains the majority of the ducts that bring digestive enzymes to the duodenum. Below and around this is the pancreas area, with the larger head located on the right foot and the tail on the left foot. The less important tail of the pancreas is located on the left foot. If there are more acute problems with the pancreas—blood sugar problems, parasites, or reflux of the duodenum into the pancreas—the pancreas will feel full, soft, and sore. Chronic conditions will show as hardness and a deep pain.

The reproductive area, for the ovaries and upper fallopian tube and the testes, is located on the outside of the heel, halfway between the lateral malleolus and the back corner of the heel. You will usually feel anything from a bead to a large area of congestion in this area. A bead indicates local irritation of the ovary or testicle; congestion usually indicates adhesion and general chronic inflammation around the ovary (or testicle, although this is much less common).

The uterus/prostate area is located on the inside of the heel, halfway between the medial meniscus and the back corner of the heel (just as the ovary/testis area was on the outer heel). This area is often tight and sore. You can also work on the lower fallopian tube/vas deferens area by working between here and the medial meniscus.

D. HEART

The heart area is located on the ball of the foot, between the bones of the first and second toes. It is larger on the left foot. If there are heart problems, this area will feel either tight and gristly, showing stress, or full, showing stagnation and congestion. Massage fully.

E. DIGESTIVE SYSTEM

STOMACH

The stomach area is located just under the ball of the foot under the first toe, the upper stomach on the left foot and the lower stomach (and duodenum) on the right foot.

Chronic inflammation of the upper stomach will appear in the stomach area on the left foot, as a gristly, "full" quality. Hiatal hernia (when the top of the stomach attempts to go up through the hole in the diaphragm) or irritation of the esophagus (where it passes through the diaphragm) will show up as a tight knot tucked under the first metatarsal bone of the left foot.

The stomach area on the right foot shows the lower stomach and duodenum, with the half on the medial (arch) side being the lower stomach and the lateral half (outside) the duodenum. If the duodenum is tight, especially with a "cable" running vertically through it, there is irritation of the duodenum from the liver discharging into it. This is a good indicator of liver problems or excessive toxicity, possibly from toxic exposures, allergens, or an internal imbalance.

SMALL INTESTINES

The small intestines are in the center of the lower arch, surrounded by the large intestine area on the top and outside and the kidney/ureter tube/bladder on the inside. Find the kidney area (as described above), then move a small finger out and down from there. This is the upper medial corner of the small intestine area. From here, massage the entire area across to near the edge of the outside of the foot and down to a finger above the calcaneus (heel bone) area. You will be able to feel the edges of the area; there will be a change in the quality of the muscular tissue. Next, repeat the small intestine massage on the opposite foot.

Now repeat the entire process of treatment on the left foot, remembering that the spleen replaces the liver, and that there are differences between the organs on each side.

Complete your treatment by massaging the entire foot, twisting and flexing it as though you were squeezing out a sponge, again without causing pain. End by vigorously rubbing the bottoms and the tops of both feet.

Reflexology is an important part of any acupressure treatment. If it is done gently but thoroughly, it can be both relaxing and healing for the client.

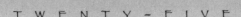

TWENTY-FIVE

The Five Elements

Over three thousand years ago, Chinese sages created a unified approach to health and healing. This all-embracing approach came to be known as the theory of the Five Elements, one of the primary tools the Chinese used to reveal and understand the implicit secrets of life. Everything from healing to agriculture is explicable through the use of yin and yang and the Five Element theory. Today, it is the basis of most Chinese medicine and central to the practice of Integrative Acupressure. It is a diagnostic tool and, at the same time, a therapeutic tool. It instructs the practitioner both on how to recognize a person's underlying imbalances and on what to do to restore health.

Nothing in the West is comparable, especially since Western medicine has yet to create a holistic understanding of the human body. To understand the Five Elements, we must understand, first, the unity between human beings and nature, and second, the unity of the body, mind, and spirit. In fact, it is all one unity—from the furthest reaches of the cosmos to the inner workings of the human cell. All is created and guided by an underlying life force, which itself manifests in the physical world as yin and yang. To the Chinese, yin and yang and the Five Elements reflect the inherent order of all things. Like gravity, this order is implicit in all phenomena, for every aspect of life. Once you begin to apply yin and yang and the Five Elements to daily life—especially to questions of sickness and healing—you will begin to see how immensely practical and revealing these two tools really are.

The Five Element theory makes yin and yang explicit, more applicable to specific situations, and therefore more practical, especially in healing. It reveals to the practitioner his or her client's underlying imbalances, the actual causes of disease; it then guides the healer in how to restore balance through the use of acupressure, proper diet, herbs, and other health-enhancing applications.

The Five Element theory is both flexible and precise. It can be used to discern virtually any type of health condition. At the same time, it is a guide to understanding every type of symptom. The meaning of everything from a pain in a specific location, to the color of the skin, to the relative warmth of the body, to the hours of the day that symptoms appear—all of this and more is revealed by the Five Element theory. The model of the Five Elements utilized by Integrative Acupressure is able to reveal a person's deepest, most constitutional imbalance.

THE FIVE MOVEMENTS OF CHANGE

The Chinese expression for the Five Elements is *Wu Xing*, which literally means "five movements." The original translation of *Wu Xing* to "five elements" by Western scholars was unfortunate, because people immediately categorized the system as a primitive understanding of nature. Western scholars thought that Chinese medicine was based on the false belief that there were only five elements in nature. Since this interpretation couldn't possibly be correct, how could Chinese medicine have value, they conjectured, since it was based upon a false notion. Also, many people associated the Five Element theory with the Greek "four elements," which further confused people and prevented a deeper understanding of the Chinese system. Thus, acupuncture, acupressure, meridian theory, and Chinese medicinal techniques were all regarded as primitive hokum. This misunderstanding was a disservice not only to Chinese medicine, but to people the world over, because we have long neglected a healing system that can contribute to the well-being of us all.

In fact, the Chinese regard the "five movements" as five stages of change. Each movement, each stage, is a specific state in the ongoing process of change. Thus, all change—whether it is in the human body or in the natural environment—is an orderly process that proceeds through five phases. Not only can each phase be understood, but it can be adapted to in order to bring about health and harmony with the larger force of life.

THE FIVE ELEMENTS AND THE SEASONS

In its broadest application, the theory of the Five Elements describes how change occurs—or how yin changes into yang, and back again—in five distinct stages. Each stage reveals the underlying character and nature of the forces that are currently shaping the thing in question—whether it is our health, or the seasons, or any other aspect of life to which we are applying the Five Element theory.

Each of the five stages within the Five Element theory is unique, yet multifaceted in its character. Each stage is so distinct, in fact, that it cannot be mistaken for another stage. Consequently, when one or another stage manifests in, say, the seasonal cycle, or in a health condition, the trained practitioner recognizes it and knows what to do in the face of these conditions—simply because each stage is so well defined and understandable within the Five Element theory. In effect, knowledge of the Five Elements acts as a kind of guide or teacher, informing us of how to cope with a specific condition.

To understand the Five Elements, and each stage within the system, we must begin by studying nature, and particularly the seasonal cycle. The Chinese maintained that the life force is most clearly revealed in nature, and that the five stages of change are most clearly revealed in the seasons of the year. For example, the most expansive stage is summer—when the life force is rising through the trunks of plants and trees and flowing into their limbs to create lush leaves, bright flowers, and fruit. The sun is high in the sky and directly overhead, pouring down its fiery and life-supportive energies. Indeed, it is as if a warm and colorful fire filled the plants, the trees, and the air itself.

In winter, the opposite stage is in evidence: the life force has withdrawn and is hidden below ground. The sun is weak and watery. There is a sense of rest, of waiting, and of gathering energy for the coming spring. From time to time, the earth is covered with frozen water in the form of snow, and, in the air, tiny crystals of water descend peacefully to create a soft intimacy and restfulness.

Spring is a miracle of renewal. The life force now awakens and stretches upward and all things are shaken with the tremors of new life. It is a rising energy best described by the rebirth of the trees. Various lengths of the small branches are bursting with the sap of new life. Eventually, this powerful life force bursts forth with green blossoms, which quickly become leaves.

The fall, of course, represents the opposite of the living tree: the life force that was so powerful in spring and summer is now in retreat; it withdraws from the outer limbs of the trees, causing the leaves to wither and fall.

Meanwhile, the sun sinks lower in the horizon. There is a gray, or metallic, feeling in the air.

In addition to these four stages, or seasons, the Chinese recognized a fifth. They saw that the period just after summer had its own unique energy, or nature. We often refer to this period as "Indian summer." During this time, there is a pause, or stillness, between the fiery energy of summer and the metallic gray of autumn. Clearly, the life force had reached a plateau and even begun to descend, but not so abruptly. Late summer is calm, much like the earth itself. It holds and protects the life force while the seasons make an enormous shift from the powerful ascending energy of summer, to the descending energy that is fall. Between the two is the middle ground, the earth holding the balance, while a great seasonal revolution occurs behind the curtain of late summer. Thus, late summer is the fifth season, say the Chinese, with characteristics all its own that must be understood if we are to truly understand nature, and indeed, ourselves.

The Chinese then saw an association between each of the five seasons and five distinct elements in nature. Each season could be characterized or represented by a specific element of nature, as follows:

Summer is best represented by Fire (known as the Fire Element).

Late Summer is Earth.

Fall is Metal.

Winter is Water.

Spring is Wood.

NATURE AND THE PHYSICAL BODY

The early Chinese sages saw in this combination of seasons and metaphors a key to the mysteries of the universe. The reason was simply that each stage, or Element, represented characteristics and associations that, as you will see shortly, yields a wealth of information. Nevertheless, this was just the beginning. The Chinese took matters a great deal further. Through long study, trial and error, and exploration, the Chinese were able to associate each season and Element with a set of physical organs and systems within the human body.

They discovered that during each season, a particular set of organs was being nourished by the life force to a greater extent than the other organs. The organs themselves were manifestations of each stage of the life force. The liver, for example, came into being as an expression of the life force at

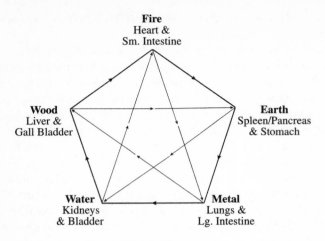

THE FIVE ELEMENTS

a certain stage within the cycle. Thus, when the life force returned to that stage in its five-phase cycle, the liver received more healing energy than, say, the large intestine.

Thus, in the Five Elements system, organs and systems were joined by their related functions, and then placed under a specific season and element.

The Elements, their seasons, and their respective organ systems are as follows:

The Fire Element is associated with summer and the heart, small intestine, and nervous system.

The Earth Element is associated with late summer and the stomach, spleen, and pancreas.

The Metal Element is associated with fall and the lungs, and large intestine.

The Water Element is associated with winter and the kidneys, bladder, and reproductive organs.

The Wood Element is associated with spring and the liver and gall bladder.

THE NOURISHING CYCLE

Just as the life force proceeds through the seasons in an orderly manner—from summer to late summer to fall, and onward—so Qi moves in the body in a pattern that corresponds to the seasonal changes. This continuous and uninterrupted flow of energy is called the *nourishing* (or *creative*) *cycle*. Essentially one set of organs is imbued with the life force and is fulfilled and sustained by Qi. Having been fully nourished, that set of organs then passes energy on to the next set of organs in the pattern. In good health, there are no blockages of Qi within the circuit. Consequently, all the organs are continuously being bathed in Qi, without diminution or excess. This nourishing cycle is as follows:

The Fire Element (the heart and small intestine) sends energy to the Earth Element (the stomach, spleen, and pancreas).

The Earth Element sends energy to the Metal Element (the lungs and large intestine).

The Metal Element sends energy to the Water Element (the kidneys, bladder, and reproductive organs).

The Water Element sends energy to the Wood Element (the liver and gall bladder).

The Wood Element sends energy to the Fire Element, which begins the cycle again.

Like the flow of electricity along integrated circuitry, the life force passes from one stage, or Element, to the next, nourishing all the organs in succession. But the life force actually provides the basis of existence for each organ. Thus, each Element is often referred to as the "mother" of the following Element, since the preceding Element provides the life force for the one that will come after it. The "Element" used to describe each stage suggests how it nourishes and creates the next. In this way, fire burns kindling (wood) and creates the soil, or earth. The earth coalesces and contracts to create metal. In order for metal to be useful, it must be melted, or turned into a liquid or watery state. Water nourishes wood. Wood nourishes fire.

This nourishing cycle of seasons, Elements, and organs is thus organized in a circle. The resulting Five Element nourishing cycle is shown in the chart on the following page.

If energy becomes blocked, or becomes excessive in any one set of the organs, the succeeding set of organs may suffer from the deficiency of Qi.

Element	Meridian	Abbr.	Sense	Body	Color	Weather	Stage	Taste
Metal	Lung	Lu	Smell	Body Hair	White	Dry	Harvest	Pungent
	Lg. Intestine	LI		Skin				Ginger
Water	Kidney	Ki	Hearing	Head Hair	Black,	Cold	Storage	Salt
	Bladder	Bl		Bones	Blue			Bland
Wood	Liver	Lv	Sight	Tendons	Green	Windy	Creation	Sour
	Gall Bladder	GB		Ligaments				
Fire	Heart	Ht	Speech	Blood	Red	Hot	Growth	Spicy
	Sm. Intestine	SI						Bitter
Earth	Spleen	Sp	Taste	Muscles	Yellow	Wet	Mature	Sweet
	Stomach	St		Lymph				

THE NOURISHING CYCLE

Treatment, then, includes moving the energy from the excessive organs (and their related meridians) to the organs and meridians where it is deficient.

A good example of this phenomenon is when a person consumes too much sugar and sweets, which stimulate the pancreas and spleen and often cause energy to become excessive in these organs. As the "mother" of the lungs and large intestine, the spleen and pancreas transport that excessive energy through the large intestine. In a strong, healthy pancreas and spleen, sweet foods typically cause the bowels to move. In this case, the Earth Element is still strong and therefore can handle the excess stimulation effectively. If this practice is repeated consistently, however, the sweet foods typically cause diarrhea. If the person continues to eat excessive sweets, the spleen and pancreas will become swollen, weak, and unable to move the energy downward into the large intestine. The result will be chronic constipation.

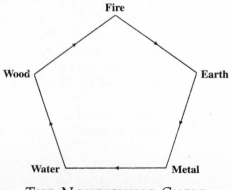

THE NOURISHING CYCLE

For many people who suffer from chronic constipation, the origin of the problem is not the large intestine at all (that organ is often very strong), but a weakened Earth Element, which is now unable to send energy downward to the large intestine. Without optimal Qi, the large intestine function suffers. You can say that the symptom is in the large intestine, but the cause is in the spleen and pancreas.

In this case, health is restored by reestablishing the strength of the spleen and by consistently moving the energy downward into the large intestine.

This a good example of how excessive conditions, no matter where they manifest in the body, ultimately result in stagnation. The excessive energy initially creates stimulation. The heightened activity also can create heat. But with continued stimulation, the organ begins to tire; circulation slows down because the organ simply can't handle the ongoing stimulation. Eventually, the organ becomes congested and stagnant. Once this occurs, its function has been compromised. Thus, an organ that was once overactive and fiery eventually becomes stagnant and deficient of vitality and life force.

The acupressurist recognizes this stagnant condition as yang—it is hot, full, and resistant to the touch. The organ and surrounding area may feel congested, stagnant, and impenetrable. As you may recall from the end of chapter 2, we begin here in the area of fullness and excessiveness. We then try to move that excess into this area of deficiency. Once again, we're trying to make the full places empty, the yang places more yin—or balanced. Where there is fullness and excess, we work to make it relaxed, pliable, and supple.

In general, health is created by bringing all Five Elements into balance with one another. Yet nourishing each organ and system optimally depends not just on the flow of Qi in the cyclical manner, but also on preventing—as much as possible—other organs from becoming excessive and thus pooling and hoarding energy. We must not only nourish, but limit and control the flow of Qi if we are to maintain balance. To do this, we must employ the *controlling cycle*.

THE CONTROLLING CYCLE

In the controlling cycle, organs limit or regulate their respective counterparts from holding too much Qi, or becoming excessive, thus creating deficiencies elsewhere within the system. A useful metaphor for understanding the importance of the controlling cycle is to think of the nourishing and controlling aspects of a river. A river is fed by the flow of water moving along its channel. Each part of the river is nourished with water by the previous part. However, the river is able to maintain its flow and power because it has banks that limit the flow of water at its periphery. If this limiting function of the banks fails, as it sometimes does, floods occur, and the water stops moving along its channeled path. It collects in pools and stagnates outside the banks. The controlling aspect of the Five Elements regulates the organs and maintains order within the scheme.

Thus the controlling cycle is as follows:

The Fire Element (heart and small intestine) controls the Metal Element (lungs and large intestine).

The Earth Element (stomach, spleen, and pancreas) controls the Water Element (kidneys and bladder).

The Metal Element (lungs and large intestine), controls the Wood Element (liver and gall bladder).

The Water Element (kidneys and bladder) controls the Fire Element (heart and small intestine).

The Wood Element (liver and gall bladder) controls the Earth Element (stomach, spleen and pancreas).

An easy way to remember the way the controlling cycle works is to see that fire tempers and melts metal; earth controls water, as the banks channel a river; metal chops wood; water limits and ultimately extinguishes fire; wood gathers and controls the earth.

Just as organs can become excessive through the nourishing cycle (thus causing a gathering of too much Qi in a set of organs), so, too, can health issues arise through the controlling cycle. In other words, the lungs and large intestine can limit and control the liver function to that organ's detriment. The Fire Element can excessively control the Metal Element, and so on.

A common example of problems caused through the controlling cycle is seen when kidney disorders bring on any of a variety of cardiovascular diseases. Often, kidneys can become blocked with atherosclerotic plaque. This causes the blood to back up and increase pressure within the kidneys, causing excess energy to build within the organs. The excessive kidney condition in turn can result in dramatic elevations in blood pressure, which often causes injuries to the heart and arteries, and can result in a heart attack or stroke.

If we take a look at the Five Element schematic, we note that the Water Element controls Fire. If Water becomes imbalanced and deficient—which in the case of kidney disease, it often does—Fire can become excessive. The symptoms may result in heart disease or disorders of the small intestine, but the underlying cause is kidney dysfunction. In the terms of the Five Elements, Water does not adequately control Fire.

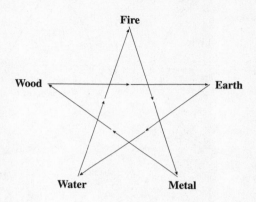

THE UNITY OF THE BODY AND MIND

When applied to the human body, the Five Element theory reveals how energy moves and changes within the body, how the life force affects each organ and system. Over centuries of use, Chinese healers developed an understanding of each Element, its respective organs, and the foods, herbs, and activities that would heal those organs.

The Chinese also developed their own precise understanding of biorhythms, or what are known today as circadian rhythms. They were able to determine at what hours a particular organ was reaching its peak functioning during the day. In other words, there is a particular two-hour period during which each organ is enriched with an optimal amount of Qi, and thus is functioning at peak performance. If there are problems with a particular organ, they often manifest as symptoms during these specific hours. For example, the ancient sages maintained that the heart receives additional Qi between the hours of eleven A.M. and one P.M. During these hours, the heart can be strengthened significantly. But if there is heart disease, the symptoms will tend to manifest in the morning hours, and become more intense as the time moves closer to eleven A.M. With increasing Qi, the organ is under increased stress, as time continues toward a peak near twelve noon. And, as any cardiologist will tell you, most heart attacks occur in the morning hours.

Just as there are peak hours, there are also low periods, during which each organ is receiving the least amount of Qi during the day. For example,

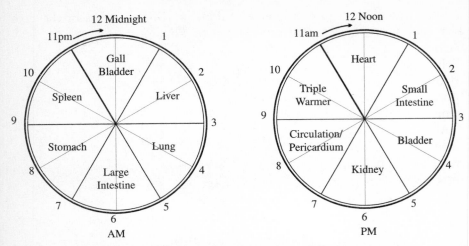

ENERGY CIRCULATION IN THE MERIDIANS
The times of highest energy in each of the twelve Organ Meridians.

the heart receives the least amount of Qi twelve hours earlier, at eleven P.M. Symptoms can manifest as well during the hours when the energy flowing to a particular organ wanes.

In order to heal individual organs, Chinese healers created acupuncture and acupressure and offered a vast armamentarium of foods, herbs, and even specific tastes that were used to restore health.

The Chinese also created a basic psychology out of the Five Element theory. As with most traditional healing systems, the Chinese system maintains that there is no separation between the mind and the body; the mind is rooted in the body. In the Oriental model, individual psychological conditions and emotions emerge in connection with the health or weakness of specific organs. When a given organ is balanced and healthy, the respective emotions associated with that organ are also balanced. Deficiency of Qi in those organs results in a deficient emotional condition. Conversely, excessive conditions result in excessive emotional states. Knowing the psychological states and the emotions related to each Element is an important means to making a diagnosis, since the excess or deficiency in any area will reveal itself in the person's behavior, character, and psychology. According to Oriental medicine, therefore, psychological health arises out of physical health, and vice versa.

Below is an overview of each Element, physical and psychological dimensions, and the foods and herbs that are meant to heal the individual organs.

• • • • •

Before I discuss the individual psychological states that correspond with each organ, it's important to note that these explanations represent extreme conditions that best illustrate the respective imbalance that I am describing. Most people with imbalances of one organ or another will exhibit less extreme symptoms, but they will fall into one of the following categories.

Also, the effect of one Element's imbalance is not isolated. The Five Element system describes the interaction between different portions of the energy cycle. If there is a deficiency in one part of the cycle, there will be a corresponding excess on the opposite side.

THE FIRE ELEMENT

The heart beats one hundred thousand times per day, and two and a half billion times in the average person's lifetime. Obviously, it beats to provide blood, immune cells, nutrition, and oxygen to every cell in the body. The small intestine draws nutrients out of our food and into the blood.

In virtually all traditional systems, the heart is associated with joy and the spirit. In Chinese medicine, the heart is called the "Palace of the Shen," or the place where the spirit resides. The Fire Element is also associated with the nervous system. Hence, all disturbances related to the heart and small intestine will affect our capacity for joy, all conditions related to our nervous systems, and our ability to manifest our true natures.

People who have a strong and balanced Fire Element have a good sense of themselves, of who they are, and consequently are able to express their inner natures with a high degree of clarity. This, of course, brings joy. Since the Fire Element rules the nervous system, people with strong Fire have sharp minds, intellectual vitality, and curiosity. Such people are able to absorb information quickly, organize it, and use it for their own purposes.

OVERACTIVE FIRE

When the energy is overactive, or excessive, in the heart and/or the small intestine, the Shen will be disturbed. The person will be highly excitable. They will laugh a lot and use laughter as a kind of cover for their nervous anxiety. There will be a tendency toward hysteria, as well. Generally, people with overactive Fire tend to exaggerate the good and the bad of situations; they overreact and all too easily become hysterical. They can burst into fits of anger or crying, they are easily "overjoyed," and all for reasons that do not always warrant such emotion. If you want to see an overactive Fire Element, just tickle a child to excess.

Depending on the degree of overactivity, the color of the person's face will range from ruddy to red. In the extreme, little capillaries will appear beneath the skin of the face. The person's movements will be jerky. The reactions will be excessive, speedy, and quick, all a reflection of a hyperactive nervous system. They talk rapidly, move rapidly, and think rapidly—often going from one thought to the next without any transition in between. You get the feeling around overactive Fire people that they are dispersing a lot of energy. They can be chaotic, disorganized, and occasionally confused. Everything seems excessive with the overactive Fire.

Actors and actresses are often overactive Fire, which makes it possible for them to get up and perform before so many people. Performers of all kinds need a high degree of Fire to burn bright and send out lots of energy to people.

All of us have experienced overactive Fire at one time or another—we've all been a bit crazy with emotion—but many people have overactive Fire conditions.

Famous examples of an overactive Fire are Robin Williams, a person whose mental speed is unrivaled by any other performer; Sammy Davis, Jr., especially when he was performing his dance routines or smoking cigarettes and pacing a room with his characteristic jerky motions; and Liza Minelli, smiling like a searchlight and thrusting her arms wide open, virtually bursting with energy.

UNDERACTIVE FIRE

Those with an underactive Fire Element have all the opposite characteristics of their overactive counterparts. The underactive Fire people are slow-moving, understated, and lack a strong sense of self. Typically, they have a flat effect. They experience little or no joy. They are often depressed, some severely so. Ironically, many people with underactive Fire Element don't even know they're depressed. They simply pass through life in a kind of haze, so bland as to be anonymous.

Underactive Fire people emphasize order and are constantly organizing themselves, very often to the point that nothing gets done. Forms and paperwork take on inordinate importance, often to the point of ritual. People with underactive Fire often lack the ability to initiate projects. They lack that fire or passion that allows them to dive headfirst into a job and give themselves entirely to the work at hand.

Well-known examples of underactive Fire include the stereotypical bureaucrat or government worker, for whom forms and paperwork are the central task, yet lead nowhere and accomplish nothing.

OTHER CHARACTERISTICS OF THE FIRE ELEMENT

The nature of the Fire Element is peak rising energy. The color associated with the Element is red. The flavors that create Fire energy are hot spices and bitter taste, such as that found in coffee.

The hours of the day when the heart is receiving its maximum Qi are eleven A.M. to one P.M. The small intestine receives its maximum Qi from one P.M. to three P.M.

VOICE DIAGNOSIS

You can tell a lot about a person's condition from the voice. Each of the Five Elements has a corresponding voice quality that reveals the health or imbalance of its related organs.

When the Fire energy is excessive, the voice will be imbued with a quality of laughter. The person's speech will likely be fast, and infused with a lot of fiery emotions. When the Fire energy is deficient, the speech will be slow and fat and devoid of emotion.

We are so used to ignoring the qualities of people's speech that it can take some work to focus and listen to a person's voice, as opposed to his or her words. Once you do, you will be amazed at how much you can learn simply by listening to qualities of voice.

Foods that enhance the Fire Element

Grains: amaranth, corn (maize, popcorn)

Beans: red lentils

Vegetables: asparagus, Brussels sprouts, chives, collard greens, endive, okra, scallions

Fruits: apricots, guavas, persimmons, raspberries, strawberries

Fish: shrimp

Others: chicory, dandelion, spices

THE EARTH ELEMENT

The stomach, spleen, and pancreas are seen as the transformers of food into Qi, and the transporters of Qi throughout the body. This role falls mostly upon the spleen, which is widely regarded in Chinese medicine as the ruler of this three-organ Element. The spleen enhances the function of the pancreas, say the Chinese.

While the spleen is not given much respect or appreciation in the West, it is among the most revered organs in the Chinese system. The spleen is said to maintain our emotional and psychological equilibrium. The spleen can be found to the left of the sternum, within the rib cage. The Chinese maintain that the spleen is highly sensitive to all types of vibration and foods. Walking along the street, your spleen feels the impact of the traffic and the noise, as well as the harmony in the environment. Even one's own voice can be soothing or disturbing to the spleen.

The Chinese maintain that because the spleen is both vulnerable and sensitive, it can be used as a barometer for our own emotional and psychological stability. If the spleen is strong and centered, the mind will be stable, as well. If the spleen is disturbed, our whole lives will be disturbed, especially the mind. A stable emotional and psychological state results in the ability to understand others (one doesn't feel threatened easily by others) and the capacity for a certain degree of empathy. Thus, the Earth Element, including the stomach, pancreas, and spleen, is associated with compassion, sensitivity, and understanding.

Compassion without excessive sympathy, empathy without a morose overidentification with another's problem—these balanced approaches to relationships are the basis for establishing and observing boundaries between oneself and others. People with a strong Earth Element are able to recognize and respect limits in relationships, while those with overactive or weak spleens tend to have trouble in these areas.

OVERACTIVE EARTH ELEMENT

People whose Earth Element is overactive tend to be overly sensitive and thus have trouble screening out the issues of the world. They can identify too easily with other people's problems, to the extent that they often feel the problems are their own. They are overly sympathetic and easily threatened by the problems of others. Indeed, overactive Earth people often feel assaulted by the world. Their hypersensitivity makes them overly sensitive to touch, easily irritated by small stimulation. A person with excessive Earth is much like a dilated pupil in the presence of excess light: the pupil should contract and prevent the light from coming in. The person with overactive Earth should shield himself from excessive stimuli; he should avoid identifying too much with other people's problems; he should be more self-protective. Instead, he lets too much of the world's problems in, like a dilated pupil, thus exposing himself excessively, and thus injuring his inner being. Thus, overactive Earth types are given to feelings of tremendous vulnerability.

As a consequence of this extreme sensitivity, many are prone to addictions of all types—whether it be sugar, alcohol, or drugs. Such addictions are used to make the overactive Earth person feel better, but of course they backfire by making the problems worse.

In any case, they are frequently overly dependent types, if not upon substances, then upon people. It is usually the overactive Earth Element that prevents a child from breaking its bond with a parent, or makes a mother overprotect a child.

A good example of an overactive Earth person is Marilyn Monroe—sweet, open, but unable to protect herself from others. Another example is the archetypal grandmother, who showers love and caring on children, but is unable to discipline or to demand strength in them.

UNDERACTIVE EARTH

The person with underactive Earth is often inattentive to his surroundings—you sometimes have to hit him over the head in order to get his attention. Here the pupil that opens to the person's inner being is contracted too much. The person can only see what is directly in front of him, and can only feel what he is forced to feel by others or by his environment.

Hence, the person with underactive Earth typically lacks sensitivity and compassion for others. A kind of tunnel vision often sets in. In younger people, underactive Earth often manifests as the perpetual student syndrome, the person who studies all day and can't seem to lift his head out of a book. In older people, underactive Earth can make them appear as tough as leather and just as insensitive. People with old-world ethics often have underactive Earth Element. They cannot understand how others cannot lift themselves up by their bootstraps and get their lives together. Hence they become hardened to the trials and troubles of humanity and hold themselves aloof from the world's suffering.

Ebenezer Scrooge is a good example of an underactive Earth.

OTHER CHARACTERISTICS OF THE EARTH ELEMENT

Like the earth itself, the nature of the Earth Element in a healthy state is great stability. The color associated with the Element is yellow, which when worn or displayed prominently in the house tends to be healing for the stomach, spleen, and pancreas.

The sound that supports the health and harmony of the Earth Element is singing and humming. People with spleen problems (excessive Earth) tend to sing and hum to themselves. Their voices tend to be sing-songy. The taste that heals the Earth Element is mild sweetness, such as from sweet vegetables and mildly sweet fruit.

The time that energy peaks for the stomach is seven A.M. to nine A.M.; spleen energy peaks between nine A.M. and eleven A.M.

Foods that enhance the Earth Element

Grain:
millet

Vegetables:
artichokes
chard
collards
sweet corn
shiitake mushrooms
parsnips
rutabagas
squash
(acorn
hubbard
buttercup
butternut
Hokkaido
pumpkin
spaghetti)

Fruits:
sweet apples
bananas
dates
figs
sweet grapes
melons
(cantaloupe,
honeydew)

sweet oranges
papayas
raisins
tangelos
tangerines

Fish:
salmon
sturgeon
swordfish
tuna

Nuts:
almonds
macadamia nuts
pecans

Sweeteners:
barley malt
rice syrup
maple syrup

Others:
anise
licorice

VOICE DIAGNOSIS

When the Earth Energy is excessive, the voice will be sweet, melodic, and even sing-song. When Earth is deficient, the voice will be flat, atonal, and lacking in feeling.

THE METAL ELEMENT

Medical experts say that if you spread out the surface area of the lungs, you'll be able to cover a tennis court. Though many people do not realize it, we breathe for energy. Without oxygen, our cells can't utilize nutrition, which means they die. Of the large intestine, *The Yellow Emperor's Classic of Internal Medicine* says the "lower intestines are like the officials who propagate the right way of living and they generate evolution and change." Meaning that if you cannot digest and eliminate a food, you shouldn't eat it. Eat only what you can digest and you will be living in the "right way."

Of course, to the Yellow Emperor, the right way of living meant more than eating the right foods: it meant being able to learn from life and then following the appropriate life for you. Being able to learn and to follow your own path means, in one sense, being able to take in what is needed and let go of what is unnecessary—clearly a metaphor for the lungs and large intestine.

In the Five Element theory, the lungs and large intestine are associated with sadness, grief, and grasping and releasing the old—whether it is food waste, carbon dioxide, or outgrown memories. These emotions and psychological conditions emerge, in part, because of the fact that the lungs and large intestine must grasp what is needed from the environment (namely oxygen, water, and nutrients) and release what is unneeded (carbon dioxide and food waste). Our capacity for letting go of negative emotions, memories and experiences is determined by the health of our lungs and large intestine. Those with a strong Metal Element tend to be balanced, accepting of life, and are able to let go of the past and move on with their lives.

OVERACTIVE METAL ELEMENT

People with overactive Metal seem to let go of everything with an ease that makes those around them shake their heads with wonder. Overactive Metal people shed relationships, jobs, homes, and commitments with little or no apparent regret, pain, or sense of loss. They simply move on to the next relationship or job or home. They have great difficulty making commitments and, consequently, are often wanderers.

Down deep, they fear commitment and they're threatened by what commitment means—namely, the possible loss of other opportunities; the distinct possibility that they may be making a bad choice in a relationship or job. They're always wondering if something better exists around the next corner. This causes them to remain cautious and reserved, though they can mask their inner feelings when the occasion requires it. For example, overactive Metal people frequently go into job interviews and force themselves to sound interested, but inside they are terrified of the commitment that the job represents, and are wondering how long they will have to stay if they get the job.

Secretly they carry a lot of sadness and grief, but they don't dare deal with it. Instead, they try to conform to the demands of others, adopting the personality that best suits the situation. They hate conflict; they'll appease virtually everyone and are constantly looking for the easiest road to peace.

Overactive Metal people tend to breathe a lot. You may notice that whenever overactive Metal people talk, they are saying relatively few words per breath. They also sigh a lot. Overall, there is a palpable lack of freshness in their appearance and manner. They often suffer from diarrhea. Many lifelong bachelors and those who are always moving from one location to the next are overactive Metal.

UNDERACTIVE METAL

Underactive Metal types are people who are stubbornly in denial of their needs and feelings, as well as the needs and feelings of others. People with an underactive Metal Element are the control freaks of the world. They regard their bodies as machines. They deny pain; they postpone pleasure. Underactive Metal people push themselves relentlessly, denying that the body needs rest or good food or play. They regard food as fuel—nothing more—and any kind will do. Usually, underactive Metal types are physically stiff in the muscles and joints. They walk with a certain military or machinelike bearing. They are also disdainful of people who listen to their bodies, who take care of themselves, and who respond to pain. They seek control over situations or relationships. They see themselves as leaders, as "real men," or "iron women."

Underactive Metal people tend to grasp hold of the past and never let go. They remember the unkind word Aunt Tillie said to them when they were six years old—and every single injustice ever done thereafter. There's very little gray in their understanding of truth: it's black and white, good guys and bad guys (of which they always find themselves among the former, never the latter). They have an aversion to change. They can easily become embittered and unforgiving.

They tend to suffer from constipation.

Those with deficient Metal tend to speak in long sentences with a single breath. Former senator Bob Dole is a good example of a person with deficient or underactive Metal.

Many of the Cold Warriors who make up the upper ranks of the Pentagon are also good examples of underactive Metal. Former Secretary of State Alexander Haig was a classic underactive Metal.

OTHER CHARACTERISTICS OF THE METAL ELEMENT

The nature of the Metal Element is strong descending energy. The color is white. People with very white faces tend to suffer from either a deficient or an excessive Metal condition.

The flavor that supports the Metal Element is cool and pungent, such as ginger root and onions.

The hours of the day when the lungs receive maximum Qi are three A.M. to five A.M.; the large intestine's peak hours are five A.M. to seven A.M.

VOICE DIAGNOSIS

When the Metal energy is excessive, the voice will be breathy, open, sighing, and slow. Many breaths are needed to say a single sentence. When Metal is deficient, the voice will be tight and closed, and the person will be able to talk for a long time on a single breath.

Foods that enhance the Metal Element

Grains:	brown rice, sweet rice, white rice, mochi
Vegetables:	cabbage, Chinese cabbage, cauliflower, celery, cucumbers, garlic, mustard greens, onions, potatoes, radishes, daikon radishes, turnips and their greens, watercress
Fish:	cod, flounder, haddock, halibut, herring, perch, scrod
Others:	dill, fennel, ginger root, horseradish, thyme

WATER ELEMENT

The Water Element, as manifested in the kidneys, bladder, adrenals, and reproductive organs, is responsible for holding the Jing, the life force in its purest and deepest essence. The Water Element gathers and disperses this purified Jing to the rest of the body. Since the kidney meridian is the deepest meridian in the body, the Jing is contained deep within us, at the center of our being. From this deep core, the Jing emerges to nourish every organ, system, and cell of the body. If the kidneys are deficient, the whole body will be tired and weak. Therefore, the Chinese have a deep reverence for the importance of rest, renewal, and the gathering of energy—especially in the act of healing.

Because it is responsible for gathering and dispersing the life force, the Water Element is associated with all issues involving survival and fear. The kidneys are also regarded as the root of the will. (The will, as we will see next, is expressed by the liver.)

Since our culture honors ceaseless progress, aggression, and advancement—the old "onward and upward"—and has little respect for gathering and renewal, we tend to burn out our kidneys. Hence, we suffer from a high incidence of kidney weakness, which usually manifests as lower back injuries, premature aging, and senility.

OVERACTIVE WATER ELEMENT

People with overactive Water Element are a distinct minority in Western culture. They have what appears to be excessive courage that is really foolhardiness. They tend to be daredevils, astronauts, thrill seekers, bungee jumpers. They are nonconformists, adventurers, and fearless. They go against the grain; they enjoy the thrill of placing their lives on the line. Only by putting themselves in a great deal of danger can overactive Water people experience feelings like exhilaration or fear. They are very thick-skinned.

The Chinese maintain that the Jing rises in adolescence, a time in life when people are most courageous and do not believe they will die. This is the reason young men are sent off to war: the rising Jing permits them to think that they won't be the one to be killed. Middle-aged men, on the other hand, experience the diminution of the Jing, and consequently believe wholeheartedly in their mortality.

Overactive Water people are also sexually very active, love to try new experiences, and are always blazing new trails. Eventually, these people can deplete their kidneys and become underactive Water. But until they do, they live life in a blaze of glory, or go down in flames.

For all of these reasons, people with overactive Water have trouble fitting into society. In fact, society does not condone overactive Water, for the simple reason that these people do not conform, and therefore are more likely to break the accepted norms for behavior, and even the law.

John Wayne and the characters he played were all overactive Water. Former British Prime Minister Margaret Thatcher and the Mercury astronauts of the 1960s were overactive Water, as are many test- and fighter-pilots. Ghenghis Khan and Eric the Red and other conquering heroes fit this mold.

UNDERACTIVE WATER

Most people in Western culture have an underactive Water Element. They experience a good deal of anxiety, nervous tension, stress, and outright fear. Survival seems to be a constant issue for underactive Water people. So, too, is the need to identify themselves, to maintain a hold on who they are in the face of new conditions or experiences. Underactive Water people have little or no faith. Consequently, they feel the need to control their environment excessively, even to the point of phobia. People who suffer from acute phobias suffer from extremely underactive Water.

When the Water Element is deficient, all the organs suffer fatigue because of the inadequacy of the Jing. The body is saying, in essence, that more rest and more gathering of energy is needed.

While most people in Western culture are to some extent underactive Water, the characters played by Woody Allen are particularly good examples of it. Chicken Little was underactive Water.

OTHER CHARACTERISTICS OF THE WATER ELEMENT

The nature of the Water Element is the beginning of great flexibility and the beginning of ascent. It is constantly moving toward its goal. The color is black, purple, and dark blue. When these colors appear on the face, it indicates a Water imbalance.

The flavor that supports the Water Element is moderately salty. Many foods of a subtle taste also support water, such as beans and root vegetables. Water is associated with the ears and hearing.

The time of day the bladder receives its maximum Qi is three P.M. to five P.M.; the kidneys' peak time is five P.M. to seven P.M.

VOICE DIAGNOSIS

When Water energy is excessive, the voice will sound rumbling, large, strong, and contained within itself, as if there is lots of power still in reserve within the voice. If Water energy is deficient, the voice will be groaning, tired, and lacking in strength.

Foods that enhance the Water Element

Grains:	barley, buckwheat
Beans:	all beans, especially adzuki

Vegetables: beets, sea vegetables (arame, dulse, hijiki, Irish moss, kelp, kombu, nori, wakame)

Fruits: blackberries, blueberries, purple grapes, black raspberries, watermelon

Fish: bluefish; caviar (crab, lobster, and scallops are also Water Element, but because these animals are scavengers that feed at the bottom of the ocean, they consume a great deal of industrial waste and heavy metals. Consequently, their flesh tends to be rich in toxins. I recommend that people eat them only on rare occasions, if at all.)

Nuts: chestnuts

Others: burdock root, pickles, salty foods (especially miso, tamari and shoyu, tekka), gomashio.

THE WOOD ELEMENT

The liver and gall bladder, which embody the Wood Element, are responsible for, among other things, the movement of blood. A great deal of the body's blood supply is contained within the liver at any one time during the day. The liver must move this enormous bulk of liquid matter into the organ and out at a consistent pace.

The liver is the primary detoxifier of the body. It is constantly confronting poisons that we take in from our food, water, and breath. It must neutralize these toxins and move them out of the organ before they can do any harm to the body. Hence, it has one of the most demanding and creative jobs within our systems.

Psychologically, the Wood Element is responsible for initiating and for expressing the will. It confronts stagnation and overcomes it. It is the source of much of our creativity. Whenever we are unable to express our creativity and will, we suffer frustration, anger, lethargy, and depression. Therefore, will, anger, and frustration are all psychological states associated with the liver and gall bladder. A balanced Wood Element is associated with a great deal of creativity and the will to express that creativity in our respective worlds.

OVERACTIVE WOOD ELEMENT

Those with an overactive Wood Element tend to be enormously creative, frustrated, artistic, and angry. They have a big aura field. Often, they fill the room with their presence when they enter. They cannot be ignored. They have strong wills. They initiate projects and are great leaders.

Overactive Wood types are also restless, explosive, and have trouble enjoying who they are. They are frequently disorderly and chaotic. They race through projects with a giant appetite and, as they're completed, look for something else to spend their enormous energy on.

A good example of the overactive Wood is Marlon Brando as Stanley Kowalski in *A Streetcar Named Desire*. Teddy Roosevelt, Carry Nation, and Katherine Hepburn are all examples of overactive Wood.

UNDERACTIVE WOOD

People whose Wood Element is underactive rarely, if ever, initiate. They lack will and a desire to take on new projects. They go slowly and steadily through life, maintaining a small profile, from which they retreat even further. They are followers, not leaders, and suffer from extreme inertia. Underactive Wood people tend to look at things in conventional ways; they lack creativity to come up with new ideas and the daring to attempt new approaches. They are therefore conventional types: going by the book and maintaining bureaucratic rules as if they were a sacred trust.

People with liver imbalances tend to form clots, cysts, and tumors easily.

OTHER CHARACTERISTICS OF THE WOOD ELEMENT

The nature of the Wood Element is strong rising energy, inspirational and relentless. The color is green. The flavor that supports the Wood Element is mildly sour.

The liver nourishes the eyes, and problems with the eyes and vision are associated with liver imbalances. The time of day when the gall bladder is receiving its maximum Qi is eleven P.M. to one A.M.; the liver's peak time is one A.M. to three A.M.

VOICE DIAGNOSIS

When the Wood Element is excessive, a person's voice will be loud and border on shouting. There will be an angry, even barking quality. The voice will seem deep and full. When Wood energy is deficient, the voice will seem empty, small, and weak.

Foods that enhance the Wood Element

Grains: oats, rye, wheat

Beans: green lentils, split peas

Vegetables: alfalfa sprouts, avocados, lima beans, string beans, broc-
              coli, carrots, lettuce, zucchini

Fruits: green apples, sour cherries, grapefruit, lemons, limes, or-
              anges, plums, quinces

Others: parsley, sauerkraut

SIGNIFICANCE OF THE ORGANS

From the point of view of Chinese medicine, the Five Element theory reveals a more profound significance to the various organs. Each organ within the body takes on larger dimensions, including emotional and psychological states, by virtue of its general biological functions. The small intestine is a good example. It must extract from food what is necessary for life and absorb it into the body. What the body doesn't need, it passes on as waste to the large intestine, for elimination from the body. The relative health and vitality of the intestine function, therefore, determines to a great extent our ability to discern what we need from life and then extract it from experience.

Similarly, the spleen is among the most revered and important of all the body's organs in Chinese medicine. It is associated with balance and harmony and digestion. The spleen passes Qi to the lungs and large intestine, and it is responsible for the smooth and orderly function of the digestive organs.

Both the lungs and the large intestine are associated with the elimination of waste products (carbon dioxide and feces, respectively). The Metal Element therefore corresponds to the body's ability to eliminate what is unnecessary to healthy life.

Although the early Chinese knew nothing of genes per se, they did understand that the Water Element holds the ancestral heritage and is responsible for passing it on to the future generations. They also maintained that the kidneys house a person's life force, or Qi, and the gifts one receives from one's ancestors. From this unique kidney Qi flow your talents, abilities, and unique characteristics, by which your life unfolds.

The liver cleanses the blood. It also makes more than one thousand enzymes that are necessary for the digestion and absorption of specific nutrients, such as iron and vitamin B_{12}. It also creates cholesterol and bile acids, used to digest fats. As much as one-quarter of the blood is held in the liver at any one time. The Chinese maintained that the liver and gall bladder could be seen as generals of the body, commanding the functions of the

Element	Meridian	Abbr.	Sense	Body	Color	Weather	Stage	Taste
Metal	Lung	Lu	Smell	Body Hair, Skin	White	Dry	Harvest	Pungent, Ginger
	Lg. Intestine	LI						
Water	Kidney	Ki	Hearing	Head Hair, Bones	Black, Blue	Cold	Storage	Salt, Bland
	Bladder	Bl						
Wood	Liver	Lv	Sight	Tendons, Ligaments	Green	Windy	Creation	Sour
	Gall Bladder	GB						
Fire	Heart	Ht	Speech	Blood	Red	Hot	Growth	Spicy, Bitter
	Sm. Intestine	SI						
Earth	Spleen	Sp	Taste	Muscles, Lymph	Yellow	Wet	Mature	Sweet
	Stomach	St						

The Five Element Associations

inner army of organs, systems, and cells. Because the liver provides so many enzymes that are essential to so many vital functions, the liver acts like a commander and chief of the body, providing its orders through its many chemical and enzymatic messengers. Among the associations assigned to the liver, therefore, is overall order and the capacity to maintain order in one's life.

As you come to understand and utilize the Five Element theory, you will see its limitless versatility and its ability to function as a lens through which a person's underlying condition can be seen with great clarity. You will also use the Five Element theory to guide you in your efforts to help yourself and your clients restore balance and health in all aspects of life.

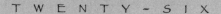

TWENTY-SIX

Chinese Diagnosis

*All of us perform our own ver-*sions of Chinese diagnosis, though we don't refer to it as such, and perhaps we don't even know we're doing it. Daily, we encounter people whose faces, body postures, and behaviors inform us about their condition. For example, say you saw a man in his fifties coming toward you. You would observe: his red face, bulging eyes, and unbuttoned coat, with his shirt open at the neck. Say he's overweight but stocky and strong. You further notice a deep line between his eyebrows, big bags under his eyes, and his mouth tight and turned down. Intuitively, you would know things about this man—about his health and disposition—though you may not be able to express your perceptions fully. You might sense that he could be the angry type and you step out of his way. If you looked carefully at his face, you might say that his red face suggests that his heart is troubled, without conscious knowledge or reasoning. You could lack a vocabulary and training that would give you the intellectual foundation for your intuitive perceptions, but you would still give him plenty of room as he passed by.

A Chinese diagnostician might say that this man's condition is hot, excessive, and fiery. His liver is congested and overly hot; his heart tired and overworked; his kidneys swollen and blocked; his intestines weak. The result is that he is angry, frustrated, and probably has lots of mucus in his throat (as a consequence of his imbalanced spleen); he's out of touch with his true nature (the result of his weak heart); chronically threatened or afraid, and consequently in a posture to fight (rooted in his troubled kidneys); and loaded with un-released sadness and grief (all of which he keeps locked away in his intes-tines). He's explosive, on the verge of a heart attack or colon cancer, and needs help. Indeed, you would be wise to walk around this man.

Over several thousand years, the Chinese have evolved an intricate and highly accurate system for interpreting the outer signs of the body to un-derstand the condition of the organs within. Part of that system they called the theory of the Five Elements, which I described in the previous chapter. But the Five Element Theory is only part of the Chinese method of diag-nosis. They have many other ways to discern a person's health and inner nature, some of which I will outline in this chapter.

The primary diagnostic tools used by the Chinese are the Eight Principles; the ability to analyze the condition of the "fundamental substances" (in-cluding Qi, blood, and such things as Jing and Shen, about which there is more to come); the causes of disease; facial diagnosis; and pulse diagnosis. Let's look at all five of these areas.

THE EIGHT PRINCIPLES

The Eight Principles is an examination of the patterns of the body and a way in which to recognize a person's imbalance. They are, essentially, four pairs of opposites. Three are specific manifestations of yin and yang, while the fourth is yin and yang itself. The four pairs are:

interior and exterior

deficiency and excess

cold and heat

yin and yang

These four states actually characterize the condition of the body's Qi, or life force. Remember, from the Chinese perspective, the body is a physical manifestation of energy. Though energy is capable of great change, it also can become rooted in patterns that can endure over long periods of time and eventually give rise to illness. Still, it is energy and the Chinese focus on its effects on the physical cells, organs, and tissues.

INTERIOR AND EXTERIOR CONDITIONS

Interior patterns are generally created by internal forces, often referred to as endogenous influences. When disharmony occurs it is usually the result of chronic conditions, such as indigestion or intestinal disorders. Often, such conditions manifest as pain or discomfort in the trunk of the body, vomiting, changes in the stool or urine, high fever without symptoms of a cold, and changes in the characteristics of the tongue and the pulse.

Exterior conditions are usually caused by exposure to environmental influences—often referred to as "outside pernicious influences," or OPI's—and one's diet. An exterior pattern is created when the body's defenses are challenged by some form of an OPI. The resulting conditions are usually acute illnesses, such as colds, or severe illnesses like dysentery or malaria.

DEFICIENCY AND EXCESS PATTERNS

Deficiency, or the lack of energy, can manifest either in a specific organ or area of the body or as a body-wide condition. Deficiency means insufficient Qi, blood, or other fundamental substances. It can also mean that yin and yang are underactive, and thus do not generate the kind of vitality necessary to cause the organ to function properly. Signs of a condition of deficiency are:

frailness

weak movement

pale or sallow face

shallow breathing

pain that is relieved by pressure on the area

spontaneous sweating

copious urination or incontinence

a pale tongue with little or no coating

the feeling of weakness, emptiness, or thinness in the pulse

Excess conditions are usually caused when some external agent, or an OPI, attacks the body; when one or another function in the body becomes overactive; or when there is an obstruction that creates an excess of Qi, blood, or fluid in a particular area. Most conditions of excess will be acute. Indicators of a condition of excess are:

ponderous and forceful movement

a loud, full voice

heavy breathing

chest or abdominal pains that are aggravated by pressure

deficient urine

a thick moss or coating on the tongue

the perception that the pulse is wiry, slippery, or full

COLD AND HEAT PATTERNS

Cold conditions generally manifest when there is insufficient blood, poor circulation, or when the body is attacked by an OPI. Indicators of a condition of cold are:

slow, deliberate movement

withdrawn demeanor

white face

fear of cold

cold limbs

sleeping in a curled-up position

pain that is lessened by warmth

watery stools

clear urine

thin and clear white secretions and excretions

lack of thirst, or a desire for hot liquids

pale and swollen tongue with a white or moist coating

slow pulse

Heat conditions are caused by a heat-producing OPI (such as an illness that produces fever); hyperactivity of the body's yang functions (expanded organs such as the large intestine); or insufficient yin (contraction) or fluids leading to a comparitive excess of yang. When an expanded, or yang, organ becomes even more expanded, it can become hyperactive, which in turn can cause excess heat. Another cause is insufficient fluids within the system, which can cause inflammation and heat. Symptoms of a condition of heat are:

quick, agitated movement

delirium

talkative behavior

extroversion

red face and eyes

body that is hot to the touch (all or in part)

high fever

irritability

thirst for cold liquids

constipation

dark urine

dark, thick, and putrid secretions and excretions, such as from bowels or urine

red tongue, with yellow moss

rapid pulse

Yin and Yang Patterns

Yin and yang are general categories within which are specific characteristics, as I discussed earlier in chapter 2. When applied to diagnosis, yin and yang are used to group individual but related symptoms, to create a unified picture of a person's imbalance.

Yin patterns are combinations of symptoms and signs associated with interior, deficiency, and cold conditions. Yang patterns are symptoms and signs of exterior, excess, and heat conditions.

There are four types of refinements for general yin or yang conditions.

• *Excess yang* is a combination of excess and heat. The person's expressions tend to be forceful and rapid; usually, he or she talks rapidly, thinks fast, and moves directly toward his or her goal. This condition is also referred to as a pure yang condition.

- *Deficient yang* is a combination of deficiency and cold. The person tends to be frail and weak, as well as slow moving. This is a pure yin condition.

- *Deficient yin* is a combination of deficiency and heat, with symptoms of both. The person tends to be weak and fragile, but with rapid movements.

- *Excess yin* is a combination of excess and cold. The person tends to be forceful but slow in his or her expression and movements.

By using the Eight Principles, we can understand a great deal about a person's condition, or the condition of individual organs or tissues, and thus treat the person appropriately.

THE FUNDAMENTAL SUBSTANCES: QI, BLOOD, JING, SHEN, AND FLUIDS

The foundations of life for the Chinese are not just in material form—bones and tissues—but living energy and fluids that have specific characteristics and purposes. These energies and fluids—what the Chinese call "substances"—are the essences and carriers of life.

There are five such underlying substances: Qi, or life force; blood; Jing, a kind of amalgam of energy and fluid that is associated with one's constitution, fundamental character, and overall vitality; Shen, which is the character of one's spirit; and fluids, which are the liquid substances, such as tissue fluid and lymph, that make up the human body. Let's have a closer look at each of these.

THE ENERGY OF LIFE

Qi, also referred to as ch'i, is the life force flowing through the meridians. It is considered yang, or an expansive and expressive form of energy. Qi makes fetal development and maturation possible, as well as all physical, mental, psychological, and emotional functions and movement.

Qi warms the body and defends it from OPI's. When a person's Qi is blocked inside the body, or weakened, he or she is far more vulnerable to illness, accidents, or attack. Strong Qi is said to act as a shield from all types of threatening influences. Most martial arts are based on the belief that Qi is the true force one uses to protect oneself from attack and to overcome an opponent.

The Chinese healer distinguishes between numerous types of Qi, depending on how it is manifesting. There is Qi from food, Qi in the air, Qi from the sun, Qi related to our constitutional development and inheritance, etc.

Qi transforms food, nutrition, and the inherent Qi in food into substances that can be utilized by the body. It then transports these substances throughout the body. The body's internal Qi is responsible for distributing the Qi taken from the environment throughout the body.

Qi maintains the body's form, and consequently has the job of "containment." Qi keeps the blood in its vessels, for example, and the fluids in the organs. It prevents internal bleeding or oversecretion of fluid. It also maintains the function and physical integrity of organs. A hernia, prolapsed organ, or even excessive sweating are all examples of the breakdown of Qi, and thus the loss of physical containment and integrity.

Disorders that result from the breakdown of Qi include:

- All conditions of excess, or stagnation, caused by emotions, diet, OPI's, or traumas.

- Deficiency, emptiness, and vacuity, caused by enduring illness, old age, weak constitution, malnutrition, or excessive stress and work.

BLOOD: LIVING LIQUID

Blood, which is considered the yin counterpoint to Qi, is formed by Qi in the middle warmer. The stomach receives the food and sends the Qi on to the spleen, which then transports the Qi to the lungs. The lungs combine it with air Qi to form blood, which is transported by the heart to the body.

The relationship between the blood and Qi is very much a cycle, in which Qi creates, moves, and contains the blood, which in turn nourishes and sustains the Qi. Qi is often referred to as "the commander of blood," and blood is often called "the mother of Qi." Disorders of blood include:

- Deficient blood, a condition that arises either from insufficient blood volume (from blood loss, anemia, or diminished production due to interference) or local impairment or blockage that prevents blood from flowing to a particular area of the body. Symptoms include dizziness, palpitations, pale and lusterless complexion, colorless lips and tongue, dry skin, insomnia, dry and lifeless hair, and a thin pulse.

- Congealed or static blood, characterized either by local or general hemorrhaging or by a contusion. Congealed blood is caused by an imbalanced Qi—either too much or too little—by excessive cold or heat in the blood, or by physical impact or trauma. Symptoms of local congealed blood include painful swelling and stabbing pain in a particular area and bleeding disorders, including menstrual disorders (excessive, clotting, black). Symptoms of general congealed blood include a dark, dull complexion, cyan-purple lips and tongue, bumps on the sides of the tongue, and a thin or rough pulse.

JING

Jing, sometimes thought of as a fluid, is the most fundamental essence of one's life. It is stored in the kidneys and is the complement of Shen, or spirit. Together, the Jing and the Shen create one's vitality. Think of Jing as a liquid energy, a kind of alchemical amalgam between cellular fluid and Qi. Jing keeps you youthful, vital, and moist. It is the source of your fundamental vital energy. When there is a decrease in Jing, one becomes dried up, tired, and unproductive. Jing provides the basis for all organic, cellular life processes.

You have only a certain amount of Jing, which must serve you for your entire life. All kinds of things rob us of Jing, including poor diet, toxins in our food, excessive fear or stress, overwork, excessive loss of semen, and, for a woman, giving birth to too many children without adequate rest and recovery between births. Fortunately, you can enrich your Jing and boost its power through a health-promoting diet, which nourishes the body, especially with high-quality Qi.

There are two types of Jing:

Prenatal or congenital Jing (*Xian-tian-zhi Jing*) is created by the parents' Jing at conception. The quantity and quality of prenatal Jing is fixed at birth and determines each person's growth and development. Prenatal Jing combines with the Qi inherited at birth (called *Yuan Qi*) to determine your basic constitution.

Postnatal Jing (*Hou-tian-zhi Jing*) is responsible for the health, maintenance, and functioning of the organs. Postnatal Jing is what we experience as our underlying strength or vitality. The amount of postnatal Jing you have depends on how much energy you have left over after the organs have used what they need to function. Consequently, postnatal Jing depends heavily on lifestyle and dietary factors. Excess Jing is stored in the kidneys and is readily available to the body as the need arises.

Jing is responsible for activating the spleen and stomach to assimilate and transform food, and is the spark for every organic process in the body. Weakness or depletion of Jing causes poor assimilation and transformation of food into energy, congenital defects, late or improper maturation, premature aging or senility, and sexual or reproductive dysfunctions.

SHEN

In Chinese medicine, Qi, Jing, and Shen are considered to be the "Three Treasures." The Chinese character for Shen translates best as "spirit"; however, Shen is not associated with spirituality but rather with vitality and awareness. It is considered to be a material substance, not a spirit.

Shen is unique to human life and is associated with the force of personality, the ability to think, discriminate, and choose appropriately. It is said that "Shen is the awareness that shines out of our eyes when we are truly awake." Shen resides in the heart, the "Palace of the Shen," but each of the yin organs is said to have its own "little Shen," which is where the emotional qualities of each comes from. The quality and quantity of Shen is derived originally from the parents, but it is continually replenished and nourished by one's environment and lifestyle.

When Shen is disturbed, the mind is disturbed. Shen disharmonies range from lack of clarity and forgetfulness to unconsciousness or violent insanity.

FLUIDS

The term "fluids" encompasses all the liquid substances of the body, with the exception of the blood. These fluids lubricate, moisten, and nourish, and it includes those that are excreted from the body, such as sweat, saliva, digestive juices, urine, tears, cellular fluids, and lymph.

The fluids are of two types: liquid and humor. Liquid refers to the yang fluids, which are more watery and mobile. These are usually found on the surface of the body and in the mucous membranes; their purpose is to moisten tissues. Humor, sometimes called yin humor, refers to the more viscous fluids, which provide lubrication and nutrition.

Kidneys govern the body's water moving the clear fluid up and the turbid fluid down. It transforms surplus and waste fluids into urine, and it is responsible in part for distribution of fluid throughout the body. In addition, the kidneys warm and activate the spleen, stomach, and lung, and are essential to their proper function.

The lung, referred to as the "upper source of water," governs the downward movement and diffusion of fluid. The lung distributes moistening fluid to the muscles, connective tissues, skin, and body hair. It also assists in the production of sweat.

Fluid is the natural extension of blood. The Chinese maintain that fluid becomes blood once it has passed through the lung. In cases of extreme blood loss, there will often be signs of fluid depletion, such as thirst, insufficient urine, and dryness of the skin. It is also said that depletion of fluid can lead to depletion of blood.

THE CAUSES OF DISEASE

In traditional Chinese medicine, there are three causes of disease: environment (exogenous), emotion (endogenous), and way of life. Within these three categories, there are six environmental causes of disease, five emotional causes, and several ways to disrupt one's lifestyle to cause illness.

SIX ENVIRONMENTAL CAUSES OF ILLNESS

As the Five Element theory reveals, the Chinese see an intimate connection between nature and the human body. Indeed, many natural phenomena, such as wind and cold and heat, are used as metaphors to explain conditions within specific organs or the overall body, and thus the basis for health or illness. Also, excessive exposure to these same natural forces can injure the body and specific organs. For example, overexposure to wind can be highly disruptive to the body, say the Chinese, especially to the liver and lungs. Excessive exposure to dampness or cold or heat can injure the spleen.

The Chinese maintain that there are six natural phenomena that can be particularly injurious, and thus they are often referred to as the outside pernicious influences. They are: wind, cold, fire (or heat), damp, dryness, and summer heat. Here is an examination of some of the symptoms that arise when we are exposed excessively to one or another of these OPI's.

Wind

Excessive exposure to wind can disrupt the Qi in the head, lungs, and liver, as well as the skin and body hair. Conditions that are brought about by excessive exposure to wind usually arise quickly and can pass just as quickly. Symptoms include convulsive spasms, tremors, shaking of the head, dizziness, and migratory pain and itching.

Cold

Excessive exposure to cold temperatures or excessive consumption of foods that cool the body—such as cold foods and drinks and vegetables such as tomatoes, eggplant, peppers, and fruit—tend to cause contraction and tightness (or yin) in muscles, which in turn contract capillaries, preventing adequate circulation to the abdomen and the extremities. This results in cold in the abdomen, arms, legs, and fingers. Sometimes, pain occurs in the related joints, as well.

The related effects on the body include thin, clear discharges, such as runny nose, clear phlegm, watery vomit, frequent urination with clear urine, or clear, watery diarrhea. Overexposure to cold also brings about Qi and blood stagnation, which in the extreme can result in chronic and sometimes severe pain.

Fire (or Heat)

Conditions characterized by excessive fire are caused by prolonged exposure to heat. People prone to excess heat usually prefer to be in rooms where the temperature is cooler rather than warm. They often have an aversion to heat. Their faces are often flushed, with a reddish complexion. They often suffer from redness around the eyes, have dark urine, red tongue (sometimes with yellow fur), a rapid pulse, and chronic pain (especially headaches or joint pain).

When colds, minor illnesses, and even severe disease are caused by, or accompanied by, excess heat, the following symptoms usually are present: thick nasal mucus; thick yellow phlegm; sour, watery vomitus; murky urine; blood and pus in the stool; acute abdominal diarrhea; or foul-smelling stools, often with a burning feeling. When excess heat is prolonged, the condition becomes more extreme, resulting in damage to the fluids, dry tongue and mouth, thirst for cold fluids, and dry, hard stools. Chronic swelling of an organ is also common, particularly the swelling of the liver. Excess heat is often accompanied by a high fever.

Prolonged exposure to excess heat can also disturb the Shen, sometimes resulting in bizarre thinking, loss of perspective and reality, and deranged ideas.

Damp

Dampness is caused by long-term exposure to high humidity and damp conditions and is often accompanied by physical fatigue, heavy limbs and head, aching joints, and poor flexibility. There may be local or general stagnation or accumulation of fluids, such as edema, vaginal discharge, or weeping eczema. The spleen is particularly susceptible to the damp. When the spleen is injured by damp conditions, the person may experience loss of appetite; indigestion; feeling of pressure or oppression in the chest; heartburn; abdominal distention; thin stool; short urination with little urine; thick, slimy tongue fur; and soggy, moderate pulse.

Dryness

Conditions of dryness are caused by excessive exposure to dry weather. Symptoms include dry nostrils, nosebleeds, dry mouth, dry cracked lips, a dry tickle or sore throat, a dry cough with no phlegm, rough dry skin, and a dry tongue.

Summer Heat

Excess summer heat, caused by overexposure to sunlight and heat, can cause sunstroke, heatstroke, and related illnesses, such as encephalitis B. There are two forms of summer heat, depending on weather conditions and the degree of humidity. The first is referred to as simply summer heat, characterized by a high fever, thirst, restlessness, absence of sweat, and surging pulse. High fever will often damage Qi and fluids, engendering weakness; short, distressed, rapid breathing; and dry tongue fur.

The second form, summer heat-damp, is characterized by a recurrent fever; fatigued limbs; loss of appetite; oppression in the chest; nausea and vomiting; abnormal stool; short urination with dark urine; soggy pulse; and thick, slimy tongue fur.

FIVE EMOTIONS THAT CAUSE DISEASE

There are five emotions that—in excess—cause internal disruption of yin and yang and Qi flow, blood imbalances, and organ dysfunction. Each emotion tends to imbalance a specific organ. Following are the five emotions and the organs with which they are associated:

- Joy turning to hysteria disrupts the heart.

- Anger or frustration disrupts the liver and gall bladder.

- Preoccupation or obsession causes injury to the spleen.

- Long-standing grief or sorrow injures the lungs and large intestine.

- Chronic stress or fear injures the kidneys and bladder.

The two organs most susceptible to injuries from excessive emotion are the heart (from hysteria) and liver (from chronic anger and frustration). Damage to the heart and spirit can cause palpitations, racing of the heart, poor memory, insomnia, sorrow, or anxiety with a tendency to weep, manic agitation, or derangement. There is also often visceral agitation with frequent stretching and yawning.

Damage to the liver can result in depression, irritability, pain in the liver area, and hysteria. In women, it can create breast lumps, distention and pain in the lower abdomen, and menstrual irregularities.

LIFESTYLE FACTORS THAT CAUSE DISEASE

Diet

The primary source of illness from our lifestyles is our eating habits. The Chinese maintain that there are three primary ways in which we can potentially injure ourselves with diet:

1. Excessive ingestion of raw, cold, or unclean food.

2. Overconsumption of foods rich in fat or sugar.

3. Habitual and excessive consumption of alcohol or spicy foods.

These are the primary ways people destroy themselves with diet. Excess consumption of raw or cold foods results in a cold, empty yin condition, with all the related symptoms occurring. The practice of eating too many raw or cold foods ultimately debilitates us, robs us of vitality and Qi, and prevents the body from sustaining warmth.

Excess consumption of fat causes atherosclerosis, or cholesterol plaque in the arteries throughout the body, blocks blood, fluids, and Qi flow to organs, and ultimately results in life-threatening forms of stagnation. As fat blocks the free flow of the vital substances to organs and parts of the body, it can create heat in some areas and cold in others. In general, however, people who habitually eat excess fat have overheated and overly yang conditions.

Sugar, on the other hand, depletes Qi and results in overall weakened conditions or empty yin conditions. It robs the body of minerals and injures the spleen and the immune system. Alcohol and spicy foods also damage the spleen, liver, and heart.

Excessive Sexual and Reproductive Activity

Overindulgence in sex and giving birth to too many children without adequate recovery between births are both injurious. Both of these can drain the kidney Jing, thereby weakening the health and increasing vulnerability to disease.

Symptoms include pain in the lumbar region, seminal emissions, spiritual fatigue, general lack of strength, lassitude, and dizziness.

Lifestyle can injure the body in other ways. Overexertion damages the spleen and robs the body of Qi. Symptoms include fatigue and weakness, lassitude, yellow complexion, and emaciation.

Chinese medical practitioners have myriad other diagnostic systems that complement these preceding examples. From the face to the tongue to the pulse, these tools are discussed below.

FACIAL DIAGNOSIS

The Chinese have raised the subject of physiognomy, or the relationship between facial features and personal health and character, to a high art. It is not the purpose of this book to present a full exploration of the art of physiognomy. Instead, I would like to give an overview of the practice of facial diagnosis to strengthen one's understanding and acupressure practice.

When considering the face and its relationship to health, we want to be aware of several important features, the first of which is color.

FACIAL COLOR

All people, no matter what their race, have a normal range of skin colors that change according to their health. A person's face can be relatively pale or flushed, even gray or uncharacteristically dark, even if he or she is an African-American, American Indian, Latino, or Asian. Indeed, this system of physiognomy was developed by a race of people typically referred to as having "yellow" skin. Yet, the Chinese point out that even within their own population, there is a range of facial shades.

Therefore, whenever we speak of facial color, we must examine the relative state of that color, and other characteristics, such as the sheen of the skin, its vitality, or radiance.

Each shade of color associated with the face indicates the relative health of a particular set of organs. As we will see, numerous other features on the face also show the health of organs. Color is not the only means of diagnosis. The practitioner must combine all the information derived from the face and its many features before making an assessment.

- An excessively white face indicates weakness in the lungs, deficient Qi, or deficient yang. If it is white, lusterless, and withered, it indicates deficient blood.

- Red reflects the heart and appears with heat conditions. An excessively red face usually indicates a weak heart and disorders associated with excess heat.

- Yellow is associated with the spleen and indicates dampness or deficiency. If the yellow tends toward bright orange, the dampness is also

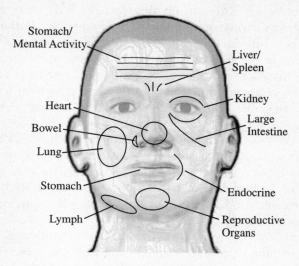

Stomach/
Mental Activity

Liver/
Spleen

Heart

Kidney

Bowel

Large
Intestine

Lung

Stomach

Endocrine

Lymph

Reproductive
Organs

FACIAL DIAGNOSIS

hot and is called yang jaundice. If pale yellow, it is cold dampness and is called yin jaundice.

- Blue-green (sometimes called qing) indicates the liver and wind and suggests stagnation or obstruction of blood and Qi (congealed blood and stagnant Qi).

- Black, or darkness, is associated with stagnant or congealed blood. Especially under the eyes, it indicates that the kidneys are deficient and weak and are not moving the blood contained within them well. This color often arises after a prolonged illness or with long-term food allergies or fatigue.

We can also look at specific parts of the face to determine which organs are most affected. Generally, short-term or acute imbalances will manifest on the surface of the face as the coloration changes described above or as rashes (indicating heat, or irritation of a specific organ). Over time, the underlying structure of the face will be affected, causing cracks or lines to form. These are helpful in determining which organs have suffered long-term stress and are a good indicator of an underlying Five Element imbalance.

The forehead shows the state of the stomach, as well as the quality of mental activity. Lots of fine lines here indicate a more precise, intellectual bent, whereas a few deeper lines show a more artistic or emotional tendency. Pimples or excessive oil on the forehead indicates the stomach is weak and contains excessive amounts of fats, especially in the duodenum.

The space between the eyebrows indicates the condition of the liver and spleen. One line in the middle indicates a long-term spleen imbalance; two lines the same distance from the center and of the same length indicate liver imbalance. If there are two lines, but not the same length, or if one is longer and closer to the center than the other, this indicates both liver and spleen imbalance.

The tip of the nose indicates the condition of the heart. A bulbous nose reveals a tendency toward a swollen heart, and a sharp, pointed nose a tendency toward hypertension. A red nose indicates stress to the heart.

The sides of the nostrils show the condition of the bowel, or intestine. Redness or broken blood vessels here suggest long-term stress, either physical or emotional, affecting the large intestine.

The areas around the eyes show the state of the kidneys. Darkness indicates stress or fatigue; puffiness under or around the eyes suggests edema and that the kidneys are unable to control and contain the fluids.

The cheeks show the condition of the lungs. You will often see sunken cheeks on smokers, as though the cheeks were empty or dried out underneath. Constant redness here shows that the lungs are constantly irritated, often because of allergies.

The lips show the condition of the stomach. The left side is the upper stomach, the right side the lower stomach and duodenum. Chapping and dry lips indicate that the stomach isn't getting supplied with enough blood, which happens in the winter and when you are under stress.

The chin shows the state of the reproductive organs. Often in adolescence, the chin gets acne, indicating heat being generated by the excessive hormones along with general heat in the blood.

Under the chin indicates the condition of the lymph. If the lymph is generally stagnant, this area will be swollen. Rashes indicate heat, or toxins that the lymphatic system is processing. These are frequently related to the digestive system, but can also be related to pathogens or toxins in the blood.

THE TONGUE

The Chinese system maintains that the condition of the whole body can be understood in any one of the parts of the body. Few organs offer such a clear insight into the overall health of the body as the tongue.

The following schematic depicts where to look on the tongue for the condition of the individual organs. Changes in color or the presence of skin eruptions in any one of the areas shown in the diagram reveals imbalances in the corresponding organs.

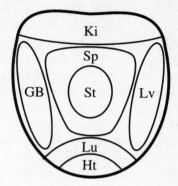

TONGUE DIAGNOSIS

Lower Warmer (back of tongue):
  Ki—Kidney, Bladder, Small Intestine, Large Intestine, Uterus

Middle Warmer (middle of tongue):
  GB—Gall Bladder
  Sp—Spleen
  St—Stomach
  Lv—Liver

Upper Warmer (front of tongue):
  Lu—Lung
  Ht—Heart

Typically, skin eruptions, such as sores, suggest a discharge from the corresponding organ. All sores typically indicate that there is stagnation and the accumulation of toxins within the organ. Red pimples reveal that the organ is overworked and stressed; there is blood accumulation, rapid circulation, and excess heat in the organ. Two conditions are specific to the tongue: the coating (fur or moss) and the tongue body or structure itself. The meanings of various changes in color and coating are listed below.

A normal tongue is pale red and somewhat moist. If the tongue maintains its healthy color during an illness, the prognosis is good. A pale tongue typically corresponds to deficient blood; the person is depleted and possibly anemic.

A red tongue reveals an extreme heat condition: that the body or a part of the body is reacting to a toxin or pathogen, is not being adequately cooled (deficient yin), or is working too hard.

A purple tongue suggests stagnation of Qi and blood. This can be due to a deficiency of the liver's ability to "spread the blood" properly. If pale purple and moist, it is a cold condition; if reddish and dry, it is a heat condition, suggesting inadequate blood or fluids.

The coating on the tongue, or fur, is the result of a spleen imbalance. When the spleen receives the pure essence of food—or its Qi—from the stomach, some of the impure substances rises within the esophagus and settles on the tongue.

A healthy tongue fur is evenly distributed over the tongue, possibly a little thicker in the center of the tongue. It should be thin, whitish, and moist, and one should be able to see the tongue body through it. A thin fur, especially during illness, indicates spleen deficiency. A very thick fur indicates a condition of excess spleen.

A wet tongue with puddles indicates excess fluid and is usually a sign of dampness.

A dry fur that looks like sandpaper indicates excess yang or deficient fluids. A greasy tongue, like Vaseline or oil, is a sign of excess mucus or dampness. A pasty fur (like oil and flour mixed) indicates extreme mucus or dampness.

White fur, especially when the tongue is wet, indicates a cold condition. If it is lumpy, like cottage cheese, it signifies heat in the stomach.

A yellow fur indicates heat. If it is in the back of the tongue, it can indicate candida or intestinal disorders.

PULSE DIAGNOSIS

One of the most fundamental means of diagnosis in Chinese medicine is pulse diagnosis. The pulse is taken at the wrist, with the practitioner placing his or her index, middle, and ring fingers in precise locations along the radius bone, on the thumb-side of the wrist.

Depending on the character of the pulse, and its location on the wrist, the practitioner can determine the precise health, character, and vitality of all the body's organs.

Although a pulse can be felt at various points on the body, Chinese medicine emphasizes taking it at the radial artery near the wrist. Ideally, both patient and physician are relaxed. The *Nei Jing,* the fundamental Chinese medical text that dates back 2,500 years, suggests that the pulse be taken in the early morning, when the body is calmest. The physician places his or her middle finger up against the lower knob on the posterior side of the radius (radial eminence). The index finger will then naturally fall next to the wrist, and the middle and ring fingers will rest next to the index finger. The pulse can thus be felt in three positions on each wrist: the index finger touches the body at the first position, the middle finger touches at the second position, and the ring finger at the third position.

Chinese pulse theory reveals the condition of specific organs related to each position on the wrist. For now, we will assume that the three fingers all feel the same and that the pulse is the same on each wrist. The pulse is palpated at two levels of pressure: superficial and deep. At the first or superficial level, the skin is lightly touched; at the second depth moderate pressure is applied.

A normal or harmoniously balanced pulse is felt mainly at the middle level. Normal speed is between four and five beats per complete respiration (one inhalation and one exhalation), amounting to about seventy to seventy-five beats per minute. The quality of a normal pulse is elastic and "lively," neither hard and unyielding nor flaccid and indistinct. A normal pulse is said to be "spirited." The normal pulse may vary, however: an athlete's normal pulse may be slow; a woman's pulse is usually softer and slightly faster than a man's; children's pulses are faster than adults'; a heavy person's pulse tends to be slow and deep, while a thin person's is more superficial.

Disharmonies in the body leave a clear imprint on the pulse. Classical Chinese texts reflect a centuries-old effort to classify the basic pulses with their associated disharmonies. Though there are as many as thirty pulses that can be distinguished by experts, I provide the eighteen pulses that are most commonly felt.

TYPES OF PULSE

The first eighteen types of pulse, described below, are the most important and indicate primary disharmonies. The distinctions between pulses most commonly made by Oriental physicians are depth (the level at which the pulse is perceptible), speed, width, strength, overall shape and quality, length and rhythm.

Depth

A *floating* pulse is "higher" than normal, distinct at a light or superficial level of pressure and less perceptible when palpated at the middle and deep levels. It indicates an OPI (outside pernicious influence), suggesting that the disharmony is in the superficial parts of the body, such as the skin, large intestine, and nervous system. A floating pulse is classified as yang because its inflated and swollen nature corresponds to a primary yang characteristic.

A floating pulse frequently occurs without any other signs, suggesting an OPI. In this case, if it is also without strength, the floating pulse signifies deficient yin. This is because the pulse is active or "dancing," a sign of relative excess yang and therefore of deficient yin.

PULSE POSITION CORRESPONDENCES
The Six Pulse Positions

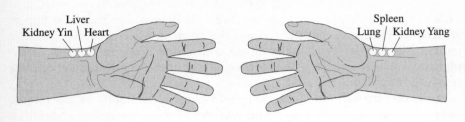

Left Wrist

	Deep Pulse	Superficial Depth
First position (index finger)	Heart	Small Intestine
Second position (middle finger)	Liver	Gall Bladder
Third position (ring finger)	Kidney Yin	Bladder

Right Wrist

	Deep Pulse	Superficial Depth
First position (index finger)	Lung	Large Intestine
Second position (middle finger)	Spleen	Stomach
Third position (ring finger)	Kidney Yang	Abdomen

A *sinking* or *deep* pulse is distinct only at the third level, when heavy pressure is applied. It indicates that the disharmony is internal or that there is obstruction, such as in the intestines, liver, or kidneys. It is accordingly classified as yin.

Speed
A *slow* pulse has fewer than four beats per respiration. It is a sign of cold retarding movement or of insufficient Qi. It is described as yin.

A *rapid* pulse has more than five beats per respiration. It indicates that heat is accelerating the movement of blood. It is accordingly a yang pulse.

Width

A *thin* pulse feels like a fine thread but is very distinct and clear. It is a sign of deficient blood, unable to fill the pulse properly. It is also often a sign of deficient Qi and is described as yin.

A *big* pulse is broad in diameter and very distinct, and it suggests excess. It is commonly felt when heat is in the stomach or intestines, or both, and is a yang pulse.

Strength

An *empty* pulse is big, but without strength. It feels weak and soft like a balloon partially filled with water. It is usually felt at the superficial level and is often slower than normal. It signifies deficient Qi and blood, and is considered a yin phenomenon.

A *full* pulse is also big, but strong, in this case pounding hard against the fingers at all three depths. It is a sign of excess and is classified as yang.

Shape

A *slippery* pulse is extremely fluid. It feels smooth, like a ball bearing covered with viscous fluid. Classical texts compare it to "feeling pearls in a porcelain basin." A contemporary Chinese physician says it "slithers like a snake." It is a sign of excess, usually of dampness or mucous. This pulse often occurs in women during pregnancy, when extra blood is needed to nourish the fetus. It is considered "yang within yin."

A *choppy* pulse is the opposite of a slippery pulse. It is uneven and rough, and sometimes irregular in strength and fullness. Chinese texts liken it to "a knife scraping bamboo or a sick silkworm eating a mulberry leaf." When this pulse is also described as being thin, it is a sign of deficient blood or deficient jing. It can also be a sign of congealed blood.

A *wiry* pulse has a taut feeling, like a guitar or violin string. It is strong, rebounds against pressure at all levels, and hits the fingers evenly. But it has no fluidity or wavelike qualities. It signifies stagnation in the body, usually related to a disharmony that impairs the flowing and spreading functions of the liver and gall bladder. It is a yang pulse.

A *tight* pulse is strong and seems to bounce from side to side like a taut rope. It is fuller and more elastic than the wiry pulse. Vibrating and urgent, it seems faster than it actually is. This pulse is associated with excess, cold, and stagnation. It is considered yang within yin.

Length

A *short* pulse does not fill the spaces under the three fingers and is usually felt in only one position. It is often a sign of deficient Qi and is classified as yin.

A *long* pulse is the opposite of a short pulse. It is perceptible beyond the first and third positions; that is, it continues to be felt closer to the hand or up toward the elbow. If it is of normal speed and strength, it is not considered a sign of disharmony. But if it is also tight and wiry, it points to excess and is considered a yang pulse.

Rhythm

The knotted, hurried, and intermittent pulses are sometimes congenital, in which case they are not necessarily signs of disharmony.

A *knotted* pulse is a slow pulse that skips beats irregularly. It is a sign of cold obstructing the Qi and blood, though it may also indicate deficient Qi, blood, or Jing. This pulse is often a sign of the heart not ruling the blood properly, and the more interruptions in rhythm, the more severe is the condition. A knotted pulse is classified as yin.

A *hurried* pulse is a rapid pulse that skips beats irregularly. It is usually a sign of heat agitating the Qi and blood, and is considered a yang pulse.

An *intermittent* pulse usually skips beats than the previous two pulses, but does so in a regular pattern. It is often associated with the heart, signifying a serious disharmony, or it can signal the exhausted state of all the organs. It is a yin pulse.

A moderate pulse is a healthy, perfectly balanced pulse normal in depth, speed, strength, and width. It is quite rare, and pulse discussions list it as a secondary condition. A patient does not have to have a perfect pulse in order for a Chinese physician to issue a clean bill of health. In fact, healthy people seldom do have it. Everyone has some type of constitutional and age-related disposition toward yin or yang disharmonies, and each person's "normal" pulse will reveal this propensity. The important thing when reading the pulse is to correspond the pulse with other signs of health or illness. Therefore, a Chinese physician will use all the tools of diagnosis before making his or her assessment of a person's health.

By combining these diagnostic tools, along with the information you derive from placing your hands on your client, you will be able to determine the person's imbalances and work on him or her accordingly. The more you use Chinese diagnosis, the more you will use it in daily life—while you are walking down the street, waiting in the checkout line in a store, or sitting on a park bench and watching people. Chinese diagnosis becomes a lifetime study, growing ever deeper the more you understand this ancient wisdom.

A Healing Diet

The essence of acupressure is that it heals by balancing the body's Qi, the vital fluids, such as blood, lymph, and Jing. Balance is restored by moving the Qi and fluids away from the places where they are excessive or stagnant; by sending additional Qi and fluids to the places where they are deficient and empty; and by releasing the tension and blockages that prevent ongoing and unencumbered circulation of these vital substances throughout the body.

All illness is caused by imbalance. Indeed, all of life's misery and pain stem from this same cause: disproportionate accumulation in certain places, with disproportionate emptiness in others. In the case of the human body, Qi and the vital fluids are the fundamental substances of life. Disorders arise when these substances become blocked and stagnant. When that happens, cells and organs are deprived of what they need most: life force and the constituents that support life, including oxygen, nutrition, and immune cells. Conversely, health and healing arise from the abundant flow of Qi and the vital fluids.

Each person controls the flow of Qi and fluids by the ways in which we think and behave. One of the most powerful behaviors for controlling Qi and the vital fluids is our daily eating habits. Our food and drink are transformed into Qi and fluids, including blood. The quality of our food determines the quality of our Qi and blood. Even more, our food determines how Qi and vital fluids flow within the body. Every time we eat a high-fat meal, for example, we block the flow of blood and Qi. Every time we eat processed, fiberless foods, we weaken the intestinal tract. Every time we eat excessively sweet or acidic foods, we weaken our spleen, an organ that, from the Chinese perspective, is critical to our health.

Whenever I work on a client, I can tell what he or she eats on a regular basis. This is not as mysterious or otherworldly as it may sound. After working on thousands of people for more than twenty years, my hands can feel whether my client is on a high-fat diet, whether he or she eats lots of animal proteins or lots of processed foods and sweets. Those who eat a greater amount of hamburgers, French fries, and other junk foods very often have layers of hard fat and tension in their tissues. That fat and tension must be worked through and gently released so that I can get to the acupressure points and meridians below. People who eat lots of sweets, processed foods, and soft dairy products often have a soft layer of fat surrounding their tissues. Very often, I find myself trying to bring up their Qi and instill this layer of soft fat with life energy, vitality, and firmness.

Those who eat diets based more on whole grains, fresh vegetables, fruit, and low-fat animal foods tend to have more supple and flexible tissues. Their Qi, meridians, and points are easier to find, and, when blocked, their points and meridians release with greater ease. It's a lot easier to restore balance and the flow of Qi in their bodies. Diet plays an essential role in all aspects of health, but especially when you are attempting to use acupressure to promote Qi flow throughout the system.

As we saw in chapter 25, discussing the Five Element theory, individual foods can provide a tonic or healing effect on specific organs. The Qi in specific whole grains, fresh vegetables, fruit, and certain animal foods enhances the function of individual organs, and thereby promotes health and healing. Food, as Hippocrates said twenty-five hundred years ago, is medicine.

The promotion of abundant Qi flow is only one way to look at the effect food has on health, however.

MALNOURISHMENT AND THE AMERICAN DIET

One of the great ironies of modern life is that we Americans are seriously malnourished. We often think of malnourishment as starvation, but it can also mean "suffering from improper nutrition," as the American Heritage Dictionary points out. Americans are starving for proper nutrition. Instead of eating what we need, we poison ourselves each day with an excess of fat, cholesterol, protein, refined foods, pesticides, chemical additives, and industrial pollutants that inadvertently wind up in our foods. The consequence is an epidemic of degenerative disease unlike any in history. The numbers of the sick and dead are numbing: nearly sixty million Americans suffer from heart and artery diseases; a million new cases of cancer are diagnosed each year, and half a million die annually from cancer; twenty-five million have osteoporosis; twelve million have diabetes; one in four adults is obese.

Despite our advanced technology and science, we rank low in the world's longevity race. According to the World Health Organization, American women rank sixteenth in longevity, living 78.6 years on average; American men are twenty-second, living to 71.6 years on average. The oldest living people on earth are the Japanese, whose women live, on average, to 82.5, and the men to 76.2. They are followed by the French.

One could make a good argument that the quality of our latter years is also inferior to many traditional societies, since so many of us suffer from porous bones that easily break, or require powerful drugs and surgery to maintain our faculties. The Japanese, Chinese, and Europeans are not nearly as medicated or operated on as we are. The vast majority of our health problems stem from a diet made up of beef, pork, eggs, butter, cheese, milk, refined flours, sugar, and artificial ingredients.

The fact is that we were never meant to eat this way. That's not a moral judgment, but the judgment of nature. Our species evolved on a diet made up primarily of vegetable foods. The people who continue to eat the way our ancestors did remain relatively free of the degenerative diseases that are so prevalent among modern cultures.

T. Colin Campbell, Ph.D., an epidemiologist from Cornell University who examined the diets and health patterns of 6,500 Chinese, found that the Chinese have extremely low rates of the common cancers: breast, colon, and prostate; they also experience low rates of heart disease, diabetes, osteoporosis, and obesity. The Chinese diet is composed mostly of vegetable foods, such as rice, leafy greens, and roots. They eat no dairy foods, but nevertheless have strong bones throughout their lives. After reporting his findings, Dr. Campbell told the *New York Times*, "We're basically a vegetarian species and should be eating a wide variety of plant foods and minimizing our intake of animal foods."

Since grains, vegetables, beans, and fruit were the most abundant foods available, the human body evolved so that it could accommodate this food efficiently. For example, because we have consumed mostly grains and vegetables, our teeth are dominated by molars. These molars and premolars are very effective for grinding grain, but lousy at tearing and masticating meat. Of our thirty-two teeth, only four are canine, and even these are rudimentary, given that they are often rounded and dull. Compare our canine teeth to the sharp, jagged teeth of a dog or cat. These animals have the perfect teeth for tearing and masticating flesh.

Our digestive tract is long and winding, similar to that of herbivores, rather than the short intestines of carnivores. Nature designed the human body to eat only minimal amounts of animal flesh and fats. Flesh is difficult to pass through our digestive system. It often remains within our intestines too long, where it putrefies and causes a cascade of problems—everything from constipation and ammonia production to polyps and cancerous tumors.

The digestive tract and the circulatory system are intimately connected, since what is absorbed through the intestines goes directly into the blood. A high-fiber diet rapidly moves waste through and out of the system, thus sparing the blood and blood-cleansing organs the task of having to deal with all that pollution that would otherwise make its way to cells and organs.

Conversely, a diet composed of an overabundance of red meat, dairy products, eggs, and poultry is essentially rich in fat and low in fiber, a terrible combination for both the intestines and the blood.

Fat is toxic for another reason: it prevents us from living in harmony with one of the fundamental laws of the body, namely, that each cell requires optimal amounts of oxygen to survive and function.

Oxygen is the first law of the human body. Of the three things we need to survive—food, water, and oxygen—we need oxygen most and we need it continuously. Once fat is absorbed by the small intestines and enters our bloodstream, it prevents blood and oxygen from flowing to cells. Cells suffocate. Some die, others mutate. For many thousands of people each day, those mutant cells become cancerous. For millions of others, the fat forms cholesterol plaques in the arteries leading to the heart and brain, eventually causing a heart attack or stroke.

Fat also triggers the production of highly unstable molecules, called free radicals, that cause our cells and tissues to decay. A certain amount of free radical formation occurs naturally as part of our immune response and aging. Our diets and lifestyles can promote additional free radical production and thereby lead to disease. These free radicals are the underlying cause of aging, wrinkles, and more than sixty diseases, including heart disease, cancer, arthritis, Alzheimer's, Parkinson's disease, and many immune deficiency illnesses. Excessive free radical formation is the underlying process that ultimately leads to a specific illness which eventually kills us.

Remarkably, certain foods contain nutrients that reduce, and for certain periods of time, stop free radical production and reestablish health to atoms, cells, and tissues. Such nutrients are called antioxidants, or free radical scavengers. Antioxidants are found in most vegetables and fruits. Scientists have also discovered that antioxidants are powerful immune boosters.

There are many antioxidants, but the three that most people know something about today are vitamins C, E, and beta carotene, the vegetable source of vitamin A. Combinations of these are found in abundance in vegetable foods, including whole grains, leafy greens, roots, squash, beans, and sea vegetables.

In addition to the commonly known antioxidants are other important free radical scavengers, including selenium, vitamin B_6, and glutathione, a substance found in whole grains, whole grain breads, fruits, and vegetables. Once we reach adulthood, our primary biological need is for energy. The most efficient fuel the body can consume is complex carbohydrates, found in whole grains, beans, vegetables, and fruit. In contrast to refined white sugar, which gives you a quick burst of energy that falls off quickly, leaving you feeling weak, nervous, and depressed, complex carbohydrates provide enduring vitality. The long molecular chains of carbohydrates found in whole grains and vegetables must be broken down slowly in the intestines; the process is methodical and steady. The result is that you feel a continual surge of energy between breakfast and lunch, lunch and dinner, dinner and bedtime.

The diet that provides optimal amounts of oxygen to our cells, boosts the immune system, slows the aging process, and provides maximum energy is one that is made up of whole grains, fresh vegetables, beans, sea vegetables, and fruit. Our problem is not so much our failure to find cures for this disease or that, but our refusal to stop poisoning ourselves each day. By recognizing and returning to our traditional human diet, we can save ourselves from the poisons that are killing millions daily.

This is one of the reasons why the U.S. Department of Agriculture came up with its new set of dietary guidelines for Americans, the so-called Food Guide Pyramid, because all the science supports a plant-based diet as the foundation of good health. In its new guidelines, the USDA now recommends that Americans eat between six and eleven servings of a whole grain food per day, such as brown rice, whole wheat, barley, millet, oats, whole grain bread (one slice equals a single serving), whole cereals, and whole grain pasta. In addition, USDA scientists urge people to eat at least three to five servings of vegetables per day, and at least two to four servings of fruit. In other words, the diet they recommend is dominated by plant foods. At the very top of the pyramid are the foods that the scientists say we should eat only "sparingly." Those are the foods rich in fat, such as red meat, whole dairy products, and eggs. Also at the top of the pyramid are foods rich in sugar and oil.

Virtually all of the science on nutrition and health urges us to go back to the diet we evolved on, a regimen based largely on plant foods and low-fat animal products. Therefore, I recommend that people eat a diet made up largely of the following foods:

- *Whole grains,* such as brown rice, barley, millet, whole wheat, corn, oats, and buckwheat; also pastas and whole grain breads. These foods are rich in complex carbohydrates that provide long-lasting energy; they also provide an abundance of fiber and nutrition, including protein, minerals, and vitamins, including the antioxidant vitamin E.

Recommendation: at least two servings of a whole grain or pasta daily.

- *Green and leafy vegetables,* including asparagus, broccoli, Brussels sprouts, cabbage, celery, Chinese cabbage, collard greens, dandelion greens, endive, escarole, kale, kohlrabi, leeks, mustard greens, scallions, string beans, and watercress. There is no greater source of nutrition and fiber on the planet than green, leafy, and root vegetables. They are the primary source of vitamins, minerals, antioxidants, and immune-boosting and cancer-fighting substances available to humans.

Recommendation: at least three servings of a green or leafy vegetable per day.

- *Roots and round vegetables,* such as burdock, carrots, cucumber, lotus, parsnip, potato, okra, squash (acorn, butternut, buttercup, Hokkaido, hubbard, pumpkin, and yellow squash), onions, rutabaga, turnip, sweet potato, and yams, just to name a few.

Recommendation: at least one serving of a root vegetable per day.

- *Beans,* including adzuki, black beans, black-eyed peas, chickpeas, kidney beans, lima beans, lentils, navy beans, pinto beans, and soybeans. Also included in the bean category are tofu, tempeh, and natto (a fermented soybean condiment). Beans provide an abundance of chemicals called phytoestrogens, or plant-estrogens, that protect men and women against hormone-dependent cancer, especially breast cancer in the case of women.

Recommendation: eat beans and bean products four to six times per week.

- *Fruit,* including apples, pears, all forms of berries, citrus fruit, and others.

Recommendations: eat fruit four to seven times per week.

- *Low-fat animal products,* such as fish, white meat of poultry, and some milk products, if desired.

Recommendation: many people have allergic reactions to dairy products, especially those who are lactose intolerant, or whose immune systems react to the proteins in milk. Scientists at Johns Hopkins University and elsewhere have established that milk proteins attach themselves to the pancreas. Once there, the immune system identifies these proteins as foreign substances and attacks them, destroying not only the proteins, but the insulin-producing cells of the pancreas (b-cells). Scientists have shown that this process results in juvenile (type 1) diabetes in sensitive children. Other research has shown that these proteins can also attach to the connective tissue, where they are attacked by immune cells. Unfortunately, the connective tissue is also attacked, causing painful joints and connective tissue disorders. Therefore, I recommend that in sensitive people, dairy products be minimized or avoided.

A PROGRAM FOR INTESTINAL AND IMMUNE HEALTH

Over the years, I have encountered people with certain disorders over and over again. Among the most common of these repeating diseases are allergies, arthritis, diabetes, chronic fatigue syndrome, and fibromyalgia. These illnesses are all related to the person's immune system, which for reasons not entirely understood attacks healthy tissue within the person's body, thus giving rise to one or another of these conditions. I have tried many programs, supplements, and acupressure to treat these conditions. Over many years of study and trial and error, I have found that these conditions very often emerge from a dysfunction of the intestinal tract, or what is now becoming known as leaky gut syndrome.

The problem, in essence, is that the environment within the intestines becomes so toxic that the intestinal walls begin to break down. When this happens, the natural barrier between the contents of the intestines and the blood becomes porous, allowing partially digested food molecules, bacteria, and pathogens to pass through to the blood. The immune system identifies these substances as foreign, or "not self," and reacts to them as potential sources of illness. As this condition becomes chronic, the immune system is continually in a state of siege; this constant immune reaction can, over time, become a chronic reaction—an allergy—to these substances.

This is where dairy, soy, and wheat allergies come from, and research is showing that it is also the source for many chronic diseases. Over time, the immune system begins to react not only to the proteins in these substances, but to the tissues in our bodies to which these substances attach themselves. The result is an array of disorders, often accompanied by inflammation and pain, arising from the immune system's attack on individual organs or joints.

I have found that a program composed of a healthy diet with the addition of digestive enzymes and probiotics can heal the digestive system, as well as prevent such disorders from arising. One of the most important components of this program is the family of probiotics, including acidophilus and bifidus.

PROBIOTICS

Probiotics are a type of dietary supplement consisting of beneficial microorganisms. These substances compete with disease-causing bacteria in the intestinal tract. By ingesting helpful or friendly bacteria, such as acidophilus, you repopulate your intestines with organisms that the body needs to break down food and assimilate nutrients. These bacteria even synthesize certain nutrients. Scientists have discovered that probiotics are essential for synthesizing B vitamins; producing lactase, the enzyme that digests milk products; cleaning the intestinal wall; producing antibacterial substances that kill disease-causing bacteria; and maintaining our natural acid-alkaline balance. Among the harmful bacteria that probiotics destroy is *candida albicans,* which creates yeast infections, or candidiasis.

Probiotics (which literally means "for life") are essential to the proper functioning of the digestive system, but they are destroyed by antibiotics, coffee and alcohol, refined foods, and nonsteroidal anti-inflammatory drugs (including aspirin, acetaminophen, ibuprofen, and other over-the-counter pain medications), among other things.

Acidophilus

Acidophilus (formally known as *Lactobacillus acidophilus*) is a species of naturally occurring intestinal bacteria. The microorganism plays an essential role in the digestion of food and the production of B vitamins, primarily in the small intestines. Supplementation helps prevent *Candida albicans* from spreading.

Bifidus

Like acidophilus, bifidobacteria (including *B. bifidum, B. infantis*, and *B. longum*) are natural inhabitants of the human intestine, primarily the large intestines. They prevent the rise of unfriendly bacteria, assist in the production of B vitamins, and increase acidity of the intestine, which is inhibitory to less desirable microorganisms. They also help infants retain nitrogen, which encourages weight gain.

Recently, the Japanese scientific community called bifidobacteria the most important of all probiotics because of their ability to prevent reabsorption of toxins (such as amines and fennels) that would otherwise weaken the liver and cause disease. Bifidobacteria kill *candida albicans*. They are the most abundant bacteria found in breast-fed human infants. In contrast, bottle-fed babies are low in bifidobacteria, as are most adults who have taken antibiotics or eaten pesticide-rich foods.

DIGESTIVE ENZYMES

Another essential aspect of this program is pancreatic digestive enzymes, which the body normally produces. These enzymes are used by the body to digest fats, carbohydrates, cellulose, protein, and milk sugars. They also kill unfriendly bacteria. In health, the body produces these enzymes in abundance. But after years of antibiotics, over-the-counter medications, an unhealthy diet, and toxic dietary constituents—including pesticides and other synthetic chemicals—the pancreas loses its ability to produce adequate quantities of these substances. Without these substances, foods are not adequately broken down and digested. Nutrients are not fully assimilated by the small intestine and the food's Qi not fully extracted and distributed by the spleen.

Symptoms that arise from this are poor digestion, gas, bloating, headaches (especially after eating), allergies, and food allergies. Many chronic degenerative diseases, such as arthritis, many cases of diabetes, chronic fatigue syndrome, fibromyalgia, and weakened immune function are also symptoms.

The antidote to this problem is to replace the lost digestive enzymes and to repopulate the intestine with friendly bacteria. Both of these goals are accomplished by taking natural digestive enzymes, derived from natural food substances, and probiotics, specifically acidophilus and bifidus.

After years of trying many types of digestive enzymes, I have found two products that work well, Cell Tech's Digestive Enzymes and Standard Process Labs' Zymex II. I believe in the near future many more high-quality products will appear on the market.

The program is simple. Take acidophilus and bifidus before breakfast in the morning, and take digestive enzymes with every meal. For the first two to four months, you should take higher levels of probiotics (four to eight capsules total of most high-quality brands). After this, you can go on a maintenance dosage of two to four capsules. I also recommend returning to the intensive protocol once a year or whenever you get sick, for at least one to two weeks. The program will greatly improve your health and the strength of your immune system.

A plant-based diet is the foundation of good health. Plants are the richest source of nutrition, fiber, immune boosters, and cancer-fighters. Such a healing diet, in combination with health-promoting supplements and ongoing acupressure, can restore the vitality and integrity to your digestive tract and overcome leaky gut syndrome. The best approach to your health is to combine these two powerful tools: healing foods and regular acupressure. If you are a professional acupressure practitioner, I urge you to gently and respectfully encourage your clients to adopt a healthy way of eating. Together, acupressure and diet can help people overcome even the most intractable health problems.

Conclusion

In this book, I have attempted to give you an understanding of Integrative Acupressure and my own approach to health and healing, an approach that is based on the "intelligence" and sensitivity in our touch as much as it is on those qualities in our mind. Acupressure, perhaps more than any other form of Chinese medicine, is a visceral approach to healing. A person carries his issues in his tissues. The mind and body become one the moment you apply your healing touch to another person's physical disorders. Do this work and watch how the person's body and mind are both healed.

All the work you do on other people is also work you do on yourself. Acupressure is a lifetime pursuit of knowledge and wisdom, and both qualities evolve only with continual self-reflection and self-improvement. A healer is only as effective as the depth of his own understanding of his life and himself. As you traverse deeper into your own issues, you naturally feel more compassion and understanding for those who come to you for help with theirs.

Many remarkable experiences await the person who takes up this practice, or who uses it for her own healing. Perhaps the greatest is the moment when your head and hands work together in perfect harmony, unencumbered by any intellectual knowledge you may have, or any judgments about what you think you "should" be doing. The practice encourages integration and growth for every practitioner. By serving as a conduit for Qi flow to another human being, you are also enriched by that energy yourself. In the course of attempting to heal others, the healer becomes healed.

Promoting health and healing in others is truly sacred work. We are working on the "Palace of the Shen," the home of the spirit and the soul. When the body and mind are out of balance, it is like looking through a dirty lens that obstructs and distorts the light of life and spirit—our own as well as others'.

This book is not a complete presentation of acupressure—no book could hold all of its secrets. There will always be new layers of understanding, paths to new knowledge, and new bodies with hidden surprises. A wise man once said that the more he knows, the more he realizes he doesn't know very much. Acupressure is a humbling pursuit, but like all experiences of humility, it is also ennobling. Applying our limited knowledge for the benefit of ourselves and others is a great endeavor, no matter how small our knowledge seems at times.

One of the unique qualities of acupressure is that it is essentially self-empowering. Each of us has the power to heal in our hands. That power is limited only by the temporary boundaries of our knowledge, self-development, and faith. But even in the face of such limitations, healing miracles await everyone who uses this practice for the benefit of others, or for themselves.

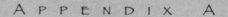

Acupressure Point Locator

The standard measurement in acupuncture and acupressure is called the *cun* or *tsun* (pronounced "soon" with a shorter "oo"). A cun is the distance from the first knuckle (nearest the fingertip) to the second knuckle on the middle finger, although it is a relative measurement and varies according to the individual and the area you are measuring.

For expedience sake, we have adopted a "fingers" method for measurement, where we start from a point or location and measure the number of fingers' width, usually starting with the index finger on the point, to the point or location we are seeking. We do not include the original location as a finger, so if your index finger is on Lu 2 and your ring finger is on Lu 1, you would count that as two fingers away.

For your information and as a way of translating (bearing in mind the relativity of both the fingers and the cun method), one cun is about equal to three fingers away, or in actuality the distance between the center of the tip of the index finger and the center of the tip of the pinky finger.

Lung Meridian

Lu 1: Alarm point. Follow the crease where the arm meets the chest up to just below the clavicle, then two fingers in (medial) just below the clavicle to Lu 2, two fingers down (inferior) to Lu 1.

Lu 3: Starting on top of the biceps, look for the furrow between the muscle fiber groups just to the outside of the top—this is the lung meridian. The other furrow just interior is the circulation/pericardium meridian. At the bottom of the deltoid where it forms a V, move forward onto the biceps to Lu 3 toward the shoulder one finger. The point is located on the muscle, not the bone.

Lu 4: Two fingers down (distal) from Lu 3.

Lu 5: On the interior of the elbow joint on the thumb side (not pinky side), two fingers away from the center.

Lu 6: Five fingers down from the elbow (Lu 5), toward the wrist.

[Lu 9, 8, 7: These points are in a row, each one finger from the last. The first finger is on Lu 9, third finger is on Lu 7.]

Lu 9: Source point. Located in the crease of the wrist in a little pocket between the head of the radius and the carpal bones, between the tendon and the inside edge of the radius bone.

Lu 8: Place your ring finger on Lu 9 and go one finger toward the elbow and your middle finger will be on Lu 8.

Lu 7: Move one finger farther toward the elbow from Lu 8, where the shaft meets the head of the radius.

Lu 10: In the middle of the thenar eminence (the thumb muscle), halfway between the knuckle and Lu 9.

Lu 11: At the outside (anterior) base of the nail on the thumb.

Large Intestine Meridian

LI 1: On the thumb side of the base of the nail on the index finger.

LI 2: Just before the third (base) knuckle, where the shaft meets the edge of the knuckle, on the edge where the top meets the side of the finger.

LI 3: Just after the base knuckle where the shaft meets the knuckle, tucked underneath.

LI 4: Source point. The traditional location is halfway up the web of the thumb, halfway between the first metacarpal of the thumb and the index finger. In Integrative Acupressure, it can also be located on the thumb-side edge of the index metacarpal where the shaft meets the knuckle.

LI 5: In the crease of the wrist in a spot called the "snuff box" (the depression formed between two tendons when the thumb is extended out and back).

LI 6: Five fingers up from LI 5 on the edge of the top of the radius.

LI 7: Two fingers from LI 6.

[LI 8, 9, and 10 are located in a row one finger apart.]

LI 8: Three fingers from LI 7.

LI 9: One finger toward the elbow from LI 8.

LI 10: One finger toward the elbow from LI 9. Also, find LI 11 and, placing your index finger on LI 11, go back two fingers to LI 10.

LI 11: Hold your arm as if it were in a sling, then follow across on top (superior) of the forearm (radius) toward the elbow until you reach the elbow joint (where the radius meets the humerus). Go back one finger and press down into the radius to find LI 11.

LI 12: Up and diagonally out two fingers from LI 11.

LI 13: Three fingers up from LI 12.

LI 14: Follow the deltoid muscle down from the top of the shoulder joint; LI 14 is located on the bottom inside corner of the V shape of the deltoid.

LI 15: At the top of the shoulder. Follow the clavicle all the way out to the bump with a sharp point (the front of the acromion of the scapula). Go just to the inside (medial) between shaft and bump (the acromioclavicular joint).

[The meridian continues over the shoulder and goes out to meet the spine at GV 14, and then goes to the scapula.]

LI 16: Follow along the top of the spine of the scapula (it feels like a thin bone extending across the scapula from the lower inside to the upper out-side). Go out toward the shoulder as far as you can and still be in the soft area between the scapula and the clavicle, just before they meet. Press into the flesh there.

[The meridian then goes to the spine between the 2nd and 3rd thoracic vertebrae and loops over to the front of the neck.]

LI 17: Find the medial tip (horn) of the clavicle and go two fingers out along the top of the clavicle, then two fingers up. You will be behind the sternocleidomastoid (SCM) muscle.

LI 18: Two fingers up from LI 17 along the back of the SCM.

LI 19: At the outer base of the nostril.

LI 20: Less than a finger up from LI 19 on the outside of the nostril.

STOMACH MERIDIAN

St 1: On a line directly below the pupil on the flat of the bone at the orbit (the area of bone on the edge of the eye socket).

St 2: One finger down from St 1.

St 3: Directly below St 2, even with the bottom of the nose, right under and a little to the inside of the edge of the cheekbone.

St 4: At the corner of the lips.

St 5: Find the back corner of the jaw, go anterior four fingers on the front edge of the lower jaw (mandible), to a little space between the muscles.

St 6: Starting from the back corner of the jaw, go up one finger and anterior one finger onto the belly of the masseter muscle.

St 7: Two fingers in front of the center of the ear, just below the zygomatic arch (bone extending from the cheekbone to the ear).

St 8: On the corner of the hairline, three fingers posterior to the corner of the eye and up five fingers.

St 9: At the pulse point on the neck where the neck, esophagus, and underside of the chin meet.

St 10: Halfway between St 9 and 11 on the thyroid gland (three fingers down from St 9).

St 11: On top of the clavicle, one finger lateral (out) to the point of the inner point of the clavicle (the "horn"), where the shaft meets the edge of the horn.

St 12: Two fingers lateral to St 11 on top of the clavicle. If your index finger is on the horn of the clavicle, it is located above the clavicle out by the pinky finger.

St 13: Just below St 12 under the clavicle.

St 14: One finger below St 13.

[St 15–18 are evenly spaced in the intercostal spaces moving down to and just below the nipple on men; they can be found either on the breast, evenly spaced to and past the nipple on women, or they can be located and massaged by pressing deeply between the ribs.

St 15: Two fingers (one rib) down from St 14.

St 16: Two fingers down from St 15.

St 17: On the nipple.

St 18: Just under the rib below the nipple.

[From here, the meridian extends diagonally down and in (medial).]

St 19: On the inner edge of the rib cage. Place the four fingers of both hands together in a horizontal line with the index fingers touching and the pinky fingers at the outside, and go up as far as this line fits below the sternum (where the edge of the rib cage is four fingers from the midline.) Where your pinky fingers touch the rib cage is St 19.

St 20–24: A tight finger apart from each other extending down from St 19.

St 25: Three fingers out from the navel.

St 26: Two fingers down from St 25.

St 26–29: Run downward, evenly spaced around one and a half fingers from each other. St 29 is one finger above St 30.

St 30: At the top of the outside corner of the pubic bone.

St 31: Starting from St 30, measure five fingers down and six fingers lateral, a little to the side of the femur.

St 32: Up three fingers from St 35.

St 33: Up one finger from St 34.

St 34: If you drew a square around the patella (kneecap), St 34 would be located four fingers up from the top outside corner of the square.

St 35: At the outer lower corner of the patella.

St 36: Follow the outside edge of the tibia up to below the knee. You will feel a spot where the shaft begins to widen before it meets the joint (the bottom of the tibial tuberosity). Starting from here, move two fingers down and one finger out at the edge of the anterior tibialis muscle.

St 37: Down five fingers below the bottom of the tibial tuberosity.

St 38: Down three fingers from St 37.

St 39: Down two fingers from St 38.

St 40: Two fingers lateral to St 38, just outside of the anterior tibialis. Located halfway from the lateral meniscus to the top of the fibula.

St 41: If you dorsiflex your foot (pull your toes upward), St 41 is located in the crease just outside the large group of tendons.

St 42: Source point. Located halfway between St 41 and the base of the second toe.

St 43: Just before the knuckle of the second toe, between the 2nd and 3rd metacarpals.

St 44: At the base of the second toe just past the first joint at the base of the knuckle.

St 45: At the base of the lateral (outer) side of the nail on the second toe.

Spleen Meridian

Sp 1: At the medial (inner) nail base of the big toe.

Sp 2: Just distal to (out past) the base knuckle of the big toe, where the shaft and knuckle meet.

Sp 3: Source point. Just proximal to (just before) the big toe metatarsal where the shaft meets the knuckle, while pressing somewhat into the muscle underneath.

Sp 4: From Sp 3, feel along the underside of the shaft of the first metatarsal toward the heel to where the shaft meets a small bump.

Sp 5: Just anterior to the medial malleolus on the ankle crease, just posterior to the tendon.

Sp 6: Up five fingers from the peak of the malleolus, in a slight niche on the back edge of the tibia bone.

Sp 7: Behind the bone up four fingers from Sp 6.

Sp 8: Up five fingers from Sp 7, four fingers below Sp 9.

Sp 9: Feel along the back of the tibia as it approaches the knee, where the shaft meets the area where the bone spreads out into the joint, pressing into the back of the bone.

Sp 10: If you drew a square around the patella, Sp 10 would be located one finger above the upper inside corner.

Sp 11: Up seven fingers above Sp 10.

Sp 12: Just below the inguinal ligament, two fingers out from the corner of the pubic bone.

Sp 13: Just above the inguinal ligament, one wide finger above Sp 12.

Sp 14: Down four fingers from Sp 15.

Sp 15: Five fingers lateral to the navel.

Sp 16: Above Sp 15 at the edge of the rib cage, in the niche between the attachments of the 9th and 10th ribs.

Sp 17: One rib (two fingers) below Sp 18.

Sp 18: Between the 4th and 5th ribs where the front and side of the chest meet. Starting from the front of the armpit, find the rib there (4th) and go down between the ribs.

Sp 19: One rib (two fingers) above Sp 18 between the 3rd and 4th ribs.

Sp 20: Two fingers above Sp 19 between the 2nd and 3rd ribs, one finger below Lu 1.

Sp 21: Between the 6th and 7th ribs exactly on the side of rib cage. Find Sp 17 and move posteriorly three fingers and down two fingers. Feel between the ribs for a sore spot.

HEART MERIDIAN

Ht 1: Take your thumb and press it up into the opposite armpit as far as it can comfortably go. Press laterally (outward) into the top of the humerus (upper arm bone).

Ht 2: Up six fingers from Ht 3 on the humerus.

Ht 3: At the inside crease of the elbow. If you make three evenly spaced dots from the inside to the outside, Ht 3 is the pinky-side one (medial), C/P 3 is the middle, Lu 5 is on the thumb side (lateral).

Ht 4: Less than one finger from Ht 5, along same line.

Ht 5: Less than one finger from Ht 6, where the shaft meets the head of the ulna.

Ht 6: Less than one finger from Ht 7 toward elbow.

Ht 7: From the bump at the pinky-side of the hand by the wrist, go to the crease of the wrist and you'll be on a tendon. Push the tendon to one side to reach Ht 7 underneath.

Ht 8: Two-thirds of the way from the wrist crease to the end of the hand, between the 4th and 5th metatarsals.

Ht 9: On the thumb-side (medial) of the pinky nail base.

SMALL INTESTINE MERIDIAN

SI 1: At the lateral nail base of the pinky.

SI 2: Just before the base knuckle of the pinky where the top and side of the finger meet.

SI 3: Just after the base knuckle, pressing slightly underneath where the shaft and knuckle meet.

SI 4: Source point. On the outside of the hand in the niche between the 5th metacarpal and the triquetrum carpal bone, one finger from SI 5.

SI 5: In the crease of the wrist between the head of the ulna and the pisiform carpal bone.

SI 6: Two fingers from SI 5 toward the elbow and one finger medial onto the top (posterior) of the bone.

SI 7: From SI 5, move seven fingers toward the elbow at the edge of the top and side of the ulna.

SI 8: Hold your arm straight down, palm facing forward, and find the bump of the humerus on the inside of the elbow (closest to the side of the body—the medial epicondyle of the humerus). From the sharpest point of this bump, go lateral just into the niche (right over the ulnar nerve).

SI 9: Just under the teres major muscle at the lateral side of the scapula. Follow the outer side of the scapula up from below armpit level until you feel it curving laterally (outward) as it goes up; SI 9 is located where it just starts to curve, about one finger down from the bottom of the armpit.

SI 10: About three fingers up from SI 9, one finger below the spine of the scapula, four fingers from the lateral tip of the spine.

SI 11: A wide three fingers medial and two fingers down from SI 10.

SI 12: Straight up from SI 11 just above the spine of the scapula.

SI 13: Two fingers medial and one-half finger down from SI 12. Also, one wide finger down from TW 15.

SI 14: Find TW 15 at the upper inner point of the scapula (the superior angle) and move one finger medial and one-half finger up.

SI 15: Two fingers up and one finger medial to SI 14, one finger up and one finger lateral to Bl 11.

SI 16: Four fingers down and one finger posterior to SI 17.

SI 17: Just posterior to the back corner of the lower jaw, pressing medially.

SI 18: Follow the cheekbone from the nose down and over to the most inferior point (zygoma), then just behind in the niche formed by the zygoma and the zygomatic arch.

SI 19: Just anterior to the ear, one finger below the ear flap (the tragus) in front of the ear canal (TW 21 is just in front of the tragus one finger above; GB 2 is one finger below SI 19 just in front of the bottom of the ear).

BLADDER MERIDIAN

Bl 1: In the orbit (edge of the eye cavity) of the eye where the side of the nose meets the ridge below the eyebrow—point your finger through the nose toward the opposite eyebrow. This is a pituitary point.

Bl 2: On the inside of the eyebrow on the edge of the orbit in a little niche.

Bl 3: Straight above Bl 2 at the hairline.

Bl 4: Out one small finger from Bl 3. GB 15 is one small finger out from Bl 4, and is directly above the pupil of the eye.

Bl 5: One finger posterior to Bl 4.

[The meridian runs back along the head to the neck from here, a bit more than a finger away from the midline.]

Bl 6: Two fingers posterior to Bl 5.

Bl 7: Two fingers posterior to Bl 6.

Bl 8: Two fingers posterior to Bl 7, the farthest back you can go on the top of the head before starting to descend the back of the head.

Bl 9: Six fingers back from Bl 8, four fingers up from Bl 10, one finger away from the medial line.

Bl 10: At the base of the occiput, one finger out from the medial line, inside of the trapezius muscle attachment.

Bl 11: By the transverse process of the 1st thoracic. Find the space between the 1st and 2nd thoracic spinous processes, then move two fingers out. Also, it is the last point you can press directly anterior on as you move up before you fall off the top of the shoulder.

[The rest of the meridian follows down the spine by the tips of the transverse processes, between the spinous process of the vertebra listed and the one above—note that the spinous process of a vertebra is lower than its transverse process. Each point on the inner bladder channel is two fingers out from the spinous process.]

Bl 12: Below the transverse process of the 2nd thoracic, between the spinous processes of thoracic 2 and 3. Called the "Reunion of All Yang Meridians."

Bl 13: By the 3rd thoracic. Lung Shu point.

Bl 14: By the 4th thoracic. Circulation/pericardium Shu point.

Bl 15: By the 5th thoracic. Heart Shu point.

Bl 16: By the 6th thoracic. Governing Vessel Shu point.

Bl 17: By the 7th thoracic. Diaphragm Shu point.

[Between Bl 17 and Bl 18 is an extra point called the glucose point.]

Bl 18: By the 9th thoracic. Liver Shu point.

Bl 19: By the 10th thoracic. Gall bladder Shu point.

Bl 20: By the 11th thoracic. Spleen Shu point.

Bl 21: By the 12th thoracic. Stomach Shu point.

Bl 22: By the 1st lumbar. Triple Warmer Shu point, associated with the adrenal glands.

Bl 23: By the 2nd lumbar. Kidney Shu point.

Bl 24: By the 3rd lumbar. Upper lumbar Shu point.

Bl 25: By the 4th lumbar. Large intestine Shu point.

Bl 26: By the 5th lumbar. Lower lumbar Shu point.

Bl 27: By the 1st sacral. Small intestine Shu point.

Bl 28: By the 2nd sacral. Bladder Shu point.

Bl 29: By the 3rd sacral. Sacrum Shu point.

Bl 30: By the 4th sacral. Anal sphincter Shu point.

[At the bottom of the lower sacrum, the meridian zigs up to one finger outside the spinous processes on the sacrum for points Bl 31–34.]

Bl 35: At the outside of the base of the coccyx.

Bl 36: Below the sitz bone (ischial tuberosity), in the gluteal fold at the bottom of the buttock.

Bl 37: Eight fingers down from Bl 36. This is along the path of the sciatic nerve.

Bl 38: One finger up from Bl 39.

Bl 39: One finger outside Bl 40. Feel outside of Bl 40 to the tendon; Bl 39 is to the inside of the tendon.

Bl 40: To find Bl 40, bend your knee and put your thumb in back of the knee in the center, as far into the pocket created as you can comfortably go. Straighten the knee, and you will find that you are on a swelling (the popliteal crease) below a small hollow. Bl 40 is on the swelling, not in the hollow. It is located directly behind the joint.

Bl 41: Two fingers outside of Bl 12.

Bl 42: Two fingers outside of Bl 13.

Bl 43: Two fingers outside of Bl 14.

Bl 44: Two fingers outside of Bl 15.

Bl 45: Two fingers outside of Bl 16.

Bl 46: Two fingers outside of Bl 17.

Skips (extra point for blood sugar issues—marked as the glucose point in the Shu points chart).

Bl 47: Two fingers outside of Bl 18.

Bl 48: Two fingers outside of Bl 19.

Bl 49: Two fingers outside of Bl 20.

Bl 50: Two fingers outside of Bl 21.

Bl 51: Two fingers outside of Bl 22 at the bottom of the ribs.

Bl 52: Two fingers outside of Bl 23.

Bl 53: From the PSIS (posterior superior iliac spine, located just outside the top of the sacrum), move one finger out and one finger down, or move four fingers outside the 2nd spinous process on the sacrum.

Bl 54: Four fingers outside the 4th sacral spinous.

[From here, the bladder meridian goes out to GB 30 and down to meet the other branch of the meridian behind the knee at Bl 40.]

Bl 55: Two fingers down from Bl 40, which is behind the knee.

Bl 56: Four fingers down from Bl 55.

Bl 57: Three fingers down from Bl 56.

Bl 58: Move diagonally two fingers out and down from Bl 57, or feel up along the fibula outside of the Achilles tendon until you find a hollow area where the bone is more palpable, just before going on top of the muscle.

Bl 59: Four fingers below Bl 58, five fingers up from Bl 60.

Bl 60: Find the peak of the crown of the outer ankle (the lateral malleolus), and move behind between the malleolus and the Achilles tendon.

Bl 61: Find the peak of the lateral malleolus and measure halfway from there to the back corner of the heel.

Bl 62: One-half finger directly below the lateral malleolus.

Bl 63: Halfway between Bl 62 and Bl 64.

Bl 64: Source point. Feel along the outside (lateral) edge of the 5th metatarsal from the pinky toe to the posterior end where the shaft begins to widen at the head. In the niche where the shaft and head meet.

Bl 65: At the base knuckle of the pinky toe on the heel side where the shaft meets the knuckle, where the side and the top meet.

Bl 66: At the base knuckle of the pinky toe on the distal (toe) side where the shaft meets the knuckle, where the side and the top meet.

Bl 67: Outside the base of the pinky toenail.

KIDNEY MERIDIAN

Ki 1: At the solar plexus point in foot reflexology. Below the pad of the foot halfway between the front of the arch to the metatarsal of the pinky toe in the soft area behind the front pad of the foot.

[The kidney meridian goes right through the reflexology kidney point.]

Ki 2: On the side of the arch in the niche below where the first cuneiform and the navicular bones meet, just behind the kidney locator bump in reflexology.

Ki 3: Source point. Between the peak of the medial malleolus and the Achilles tendon.

Ki 4: One finger down from Ki 3 and posterior toward the Achilles tendon, pressing down into the calcaneus.

Ki 5: Halfway between the peak of the medial malleolus and the corner of the heel. The reflexology uterus or prostate point.

Ki 6: Just under the medial malleolus.

Ki 7: One finger posterior to Ki 8.

Ki 8: From Sp 6 (five fingers above the medial malleolus on the edge of the bone), go behind the bone one finger and down one finger.

Ki 9: Two fingers up from Sp 6 and three fingers behind the tibia in the fleshy area.

Ki 10: On the medial side of the knee inside Bl 40, opposite Bl 39.

Ki 11: On top of the pubic bone halfway between the center and the outside corner.

[Ki 12–21 are each one finger from the midline of the abdomen, with Ki 16 just outside of the navel and Ki 21 just below the ribs.]

Ki 12: One finger above Ki 11.

Ki 13, 14, and 15: Each is located one and a half fingers up from the previous point.

Ki 16: Outside of the navel, two fingers above Ki 15.

Ki 17: Three fingers above Ki 16.

Ki 18–21: Each is one finger above the last.

Ki 21: Just below the rib cage in a small niche.

Ki 22–26: All are located in the intercostal spaces one finger outside of the sternum.

Ki 27: From the peak of the medial tip (the "horn") of the clavicle, move down a finger and out (laterally) a finger.

CIRCULATION/PERICARDIUM MERIDIAN

C/P 1: On the rib cage one finger lateral to the nipple. Place your opposite index finger at the front of the armpit, move down three fingers to the pinky. Your pinky finger should be between the 4th and 5th ribs.

C/P 2: Three fingers down from the armpit on the interior groove of the biceps.

C/P 3: At the inside of the elbow at the center of the crease at the joint.

C/P 7: At the center of the inside wrist on the crease.

C/P 6: Three fingers up from C/P 7.

C/P 5: One wide finger up from C/P 6.

C/P 4: Three fingers up from C/P 5.

C/P 8: In the palm—feel down from the knuckles of the third and fourth fingers in the space between the 3rd and 4th metacarpal bones into the palm one finger past the knuckle.

C/P 9: At the base of the nail on the lateral (thumb side) of the middle finger.

Triple Warmer Meridian

TW 1: At the base of the nail on the pinky side of the ring finger.

TW 2: At the corner base of finger just before the base knuckle, where shaft meets knuckle.

TW 3: Just after the base knuckle as you go up the hand.

TW 4: At the center of the crease of the wrist on top of the arm, slightly to the outside of the tendons.

TW 5: Three fingers up from TW 4.

TW 6: One wide finger up from TW 5.

TW 7: One finger out on the pinky side from TW 6.

TW 8: A wide finger up from TW 6.

TW 9: Four fingers up from TW 8.

TW 10: With your arm straight, TW 10 is located just above the back point on the elbow (the olecranon process of the ulna) in the depression.

TW 11: Three fingers up from TW 10.

TW 12: Four fingers up from TW 11, on the back of the humerus bone.

TW 13: On the back of the V formed at the bottom of the deltoid muscle, which extends down from the outside of the shoulder. Three to four fingers up from TW 12.

TW 14: Feel along the spine of the scapula to the edge of shoulder (the acromion)—go under the end of the spine just to the outside of the small tendon.

TW 15: At the top of the inside corner of the scapula.

TW 16: From TW 17, move down three fingers and back a finger. Located just behind the SCM (sternocleidomastoid muscle).

TW 17: Just below the earlobe behind the jaw.

[From here, the meridian traces around the edge of the ear on the skull.]

TW 18: Two fingers up behind the ear from TW 17.

TW 19: Two fingers up behind the ear from TW 18.

TW 20: Two fingers up behind the ear from TW 19, at the top of the ear.

TW 21: Just in front of the ear flap (tragus) below the zygomatic arch.

TW 22: Up above the zygomatic arch (the bone extending from the cheekbone to the ear) and a wide finger forward from the front of the ear.

TW 23: At the outside edge of the eyebrow in a small niche.

Gall Bladder Meridian

GB 1: On the orbit near the outer corner of eye, just onto flat area of bone.

GB 2: Just in front of where the bottom of the earlobe attaches to the jaw, in a little niche on the mandible.

GB 3: On top of the zygomatic arch, three fingers forward from the ear.

[GB 4–7 are located easiest by starting from GB 8.]
GB 4: One finger up from GB 5 (three fingers above the center of the ear and three fingers forward). Also one finger lateral and one finger down from St 8.
GB 5: One finger diagonally up and forward from GB 6.
GB 6: One finger diagonally forward and up from GB 7.
GB 7: Three fingers forward and one finger down from GB 8.
GB 8: Two fingers up from the center of the ear (right above TW 20).
GB 9: From GB 8 go one finger posterior and less than one-half finger down.
GB 10: Two fingers posterior and one finger down from GB 9.
GB 11: Two fingers down and a little posterior to GB 10. Feel along the back of the mastoid bone along the temporo-occipital suture. Go up to the indentation just before you run into a bone. Also two fingers up from GB 12.
GB 12: Find the point at the bottom of the mastoid, where the SCM (sternocleidomastoid muscle) attaches. Up and behind that there is a niche where the occiput meets the mastoid.
GB 13: One finger lateral from GB 15.
GB 14: At the hollow in the forehead, halfway from the eyebrow to the hairline, above the center of the eye.
GB 15: Up four fingers from GB 14.
GB 16: Three fingers posterior to GB 15.
GB 17: Three fingers posterior to GB 16.
GB 18: Three fingers posterior to GB 17.
GB 19: Up four fingers from GB 20 just outside the bump at the midline (the external occipital protuberance).
GB 20: On the back of the head two fingers from the midline, where the trapezius attaches to the occiput, just lateral to the attachment, at the base of the skull.
GB 21: At the top of the shoulder directly below the earlobe (place where a drop of water would fall from the earlobe).
GB 22: One finger posterior and a bit up from GB 23 between the 4th and 5th ribs.
GB 23: Between 4th and 5th ribs and five fingers below the front part of the armpit.
GB 24: First, find Lv 14—move four fingers down from the sternum and laterally five fingers between the two ribs, the 7th and 8th. Go down one rib to between the 8th and 9th ribs (down and laterally diagonal) to find GB 24.
GB 25: Go to very bottom of the rib cage on the side, just one finger toward the back. Press up (superiorly) and forward.
GB 26: From the ASIS (anterior superior iliac spine—the bump on the front of the hip bone) go up three fingers.

GB 27: From the ASIS, go down one finger and medial one finger.

GB 28: Down one wide finger from GB 27.

GB 29: Just above the outer hip bone (the greater trochanter at the top of the femur).

GB 30: One-third of the way from the hip bone to the bottom of the sacrum.

GB 31: Standing with your arms at your sides, bend your fingers ninety degrees and press into the side of the leg; feel in this area for a sore spot.

GB 32: Two fingers down from GB 31.

GB 33: Just above the knee on the side of the femur where the shaft meets the joint, posterior to the tendon. Press into the bone.

GB 34: Go down to the front of the bump on the head of the fibula, just below the height of the bottom of the kneecap. GB 34 is just anterior to the bump.

GB 35: Straight back from GB 36, one finger behind the bone. Also can be located one finger forward from Bl 58.

GB 36: Up three fingers from GB 37 on the side of the fibula.

GB 37: Up two fingers from GB 38.

GB 38: Up seven fingers from the crown of the malleolus, just anterior to the fibula bone.

GB 39: Up five fingers from the peak of the crown of the ankle (the lateral malleolus).

GB 40: Just anterior to the lateral malleolus in the pocket the size of the head of your thumb.

GB 41: In the space between the 4th and 5th metatarsal bones, as far toward the ankle as you can go and still be in the space.

GB 42: Halfway between GB 41 and GB 43 on the side of the 4th metatarsal, just proximal to (before) the fourth toe knuckle.

GB 43: In the niche just distal to (beyond) the base knuckle of the fourth toe (the joint of the 4th metatarsal and the 1st phalange of the fourth toe).

GB 44: At the nail base of the fourth toe on the lateral (pinky) side.

LIVER MERIDIAN

Lv 1: At the big toe nail base, pinky side.

Lv 2: Between the first and second toes at the joint of metatarsal and the 1st phalange.

Lv 3: In the space between the 1st and 2nd metatarsals, as far proximal (toward the ankle) as you can go and still stay in the space.

Lv 4: A wide finger in front of the medial malleolus, just behind the tendon.

Lv 5: Up three fingers from Sp 6 and anterior onto the flat of the side of the tibia bone.

Lv 6: Up three fingers from Lv 5.

Lv 7: First, find Sp 9. Feel along the back of the tibia as it approaches the knee, where the shaft meets the area where the bone spreads out into the joint, pressing into the back of the bone. One finger posterior and slightly up from that is Lv 7, toward the back of the medial femoral condyle.

Lv 8: Two fingers above Lv 7 at the joint. Starting from under the patella, draw a horizontal line to the side of the knee joint. Move posterior to the back of the bones (tibia and femur).

Lv 9: Up eight fingers from Lv 8 toward the back of the inner thigh.

Lv 10: Down one finger from Lv 11.

Lv 11: Down one finger from Lv 12.

Lv 12: One wide finger inferior to (below) and one wide finger lateral to St 30, which is at the edge of the pubic bone.

Lv 13: At the side of the body just underneath the ribs, one finger forward in front of the tip of the floating rib (the 11th rib).

Lv 14: From the bottom of the sternum (not the bottom of the xiphoid process), move down four fingers and lateral four fingers to the intercostal space between the 6th and 7th ribs.

CONCEPTION VESSEL MERIDIAN

CV 1: Just in front of the anus on the perineum.

CV 2: Just above the pubic bone.

CV 3: One and a half fingers up from CV 2.

CV 4: One and a half fingers up from CV 3.

CV 5: One and a half fingers up from CV 4 (the Hara point).

CV 6: One finger up from CV 5.

CV 7: One finger up from CV 6.

CV 8: Two fingers above CV 7 in the navel.

CV 9–14: Each is a wide finger up from the last point. CV 12 is halfway between the navel and the bottom of the sternum. CV 14 is one wide finger below CV 15.

CV 15: Below the xiphoid process (tail of sternum)—be careful not to apply too much pressure to the underside of the xiphoid process, as this is a sensitive area.

CV 16: Just onto the bottom of the sternum at the base of the xiphoid process.

CV 17: Two fingers up from CV 16.

CV 18: Two fingers up from CV 17.

CV 19: Two fingers up from CV 18.

CV 20: Two tight fingers above CV 19.

CV 21: Just below the top edge of the sternum, two fingers above CV 20.

CV 22: Just above the sternum in the hollow, pressing inferiorly.
CV 23: Where the neck meets the underside of the chin.
CV 24: In the crease below the lower lip.

GOVERNING VESSEL MERIDIAN

GV 1: At the bottom tip of the coccyx.
GV 2: At the base of the coccyx, where the sacrum meets the coccyx.
GV 3: Between the spinous processes (the bony bumps you feel on the back of the vertebrae) of the 4th and 5th lumbar vertebrae, two fingers in from the large intestine Shu point.
GV 4: Between the 2nd and 3rd lumbar vertebrae—on the midline in from the kidney Shu point.
GV 5: Between lumbar 1 and 2—in from the Triple Warmer Shu point.
GV 6: Between the spinous processes of the 11th and 12th thoracic vertebrae—in from the spleen Shu point.
GV 7: Between thoracic 10 and 11—in from the gall bladder Shu point.
GV 8: Between thoracic 9 and 10—in from the liver Shu point.
GV 9: Between thoracic 7 and 8—in from the diaphragm Shu point.
GV 10: Between thoracic 6 and 7—in from the Governing Vessel Shu point.
GV 11: Between thoracic 5 and 6—in from the heart Shu point.
GV 12: Between thoracic 3 and 4—in from the lung Shu point.
GV 13: Between thoracic 1 and 2.
GV 14: Between the spinous processes of the 7th cervical vertebra and the 1st thoracic vertebra.
GV 15: At the base of the occiput.
GV 16: Just below the occipital protuberance (the bump on back of the head).
GV 17: Three fingers up from GV 16.
GV 18: Three fingers above GV 17.
GV 19: Three fingers above GV 18.
GV 20: Three fingers above GV 19. This point is on the back of the top of the head before it slopes downward.
GV 21: Three fingers forward of GV 20.
GV 22: Three fingers forward of GV 21.
GV 23: Two fingers forward of GV 22.
GV 24: One finger forward of GV 23, just one finger into the hairline.
GV 25: At the tip of the nose.
GV 26: Just below the nose.
GV 27: One-half finger below GV 26, just above the upper lip.
GV 28: Under the upper lip on the gums behind GV 27.

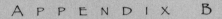

Acupressure Points for Symptom Relief

HEAD

Hair:

  falling out: GV 20; LI 11; C/P 6; Ki 13; Bl 23, 40; Lv 2, 13, 14; Sp 10; GB 20.

  prematurely grey: GV 20.

Headache: GV 15, 16, 20, 21; Bl 1, 3, 6, 11, 19, 62, 67; GB 16, 20; St 36, 40; Ht 3, 5, 6; SI 1, 4; LI 4, 5; Lu 6; TW 9, 10.

Migraine: GV 19; GB 4, 6, 20; LI 4; Lu 7.

FACE

Any problems: LI 4.

Edema: GV 26.

Itching: LI 20.

Pain: Ht 3; St 6; GB 1.

Tension: St 4.

EYES

Any problems: Bl 1, 18; GB 8, 37.

Blinking excessively: St 8.

Cataracts: LI 1; St 3; GB 3.

Conjunctivitis: Bl 1; GB 1.

Color blindness: GB 1.

Dimness: Bl 4, 23; GB 4; LI 13.

Inflammation: GB 16, 20; St 8; C/P 6.

Itching: Bl 2; TW 23; GB 14; St 1, 2, 4; LI 3.

Light sensitive: St 8.

Night blindness: GB 1, 14, 20; Bl 1, 2, 21; Lv 2; St 1, 4.

Pain: Bl 67; GB 4, 11, 14, 44; St 8; Ht 5; Bl 9.

Poor sight: GV 7, 26; Bl 21; Ht 1.

Wandering: Bl 2.

Nose

Any problems: Bl 12.

Nosebleeds: Lu 3, 4, 8, 11; LI 2, 4; Ht 6, 7; Lv 8; GV 23.

Blocked: GV 16, 20, 22, 25; GB 15, 18, 20; Bl 67; Lv 14, 20; Ht 7.

Dry: GB 39.

Pain: GB 19.

Runny: GV 21, 25; GB 20; Bl 6, 12; TW 22.

Polyps: GV 23, 25; LI 20.

Lips

Chapped: St 45; LI 8; TW 1; Lu 11.

Swollen: LI 20; Lv 3.

Mouth

Any problems: Lv 14.

Sores: CV 23; TW 1; Lu 1, 11; C/P 8.

Speech: GV 9; Bl 11, 15; St 36; GV 15.

Teeth:

   ache: GV 16; CV 24; LI 1, 4, 10; SI 5; St 4, 42, 43, 44, 45.

   decay: GB 3.

   grinding/clenching: GB 37; St 6; Bl 23; GV 16; TW 17.

Gums abscess: CV 24; GV 27; C/P 8; TW 2; SI 8; St 7; GB 9.

Tongue:
   bleeding: GB 11.
   dry: GV 27; Bl 19; Ki 4.
   swollen: CV 23; Lu 11; C/P 9; LI 7.
   inflamed: Lv 17.

EARS

Abscess: TW 21.

Blockage: SI 19.

Deafness: TW 3, 5, 7, 8, 10, 17, 21; SI 1, 3, 8, 9, 16, 17, 19; LI 1, 4, 5, 6; St 1; GB 2, 3, 10, 43; Bl 23, 63, 65.

Inflammation and pain/earache: TW 21; SI 19; GB 2; LI 4; St 7.

THROAT

Any problems: Bl 54.

Inflamed: St 12; GB 11; Lu 6.

Dry: Lu 9, 10; Ki 6.

Closing of: TW 1; LI 11.

Laryngitis: Ki 1; St 4; GV 15.

Cannot swallow: CV 20, 21; LI 17.

Swollen: GV 15, 16; CV 21, 22; TW 3, 10; Ki 3; St 11.

Tonsillitis: CV 16, 20, 21; Lu 1, 2, 6, 8; LI 1, 2, 3, 4, 6, 7; SI 6; Ht 5, 6, 7; Ki 1, 6; St 44; Bl 19; GB 20.

BRAIN

Any problems: GV and CV meridians shoulder and neck release; back of head points.

Cerebral anemia: GV 20, 21; Bl 8, 9, 10, 11; GB 19, 20, 21; GV and CV meridians.

Weakness: CV 15; GB 20.

Congestion: GV 20, 21; St 8; Lu 11; LI 1; C/P 9.

Convulsions: GV 4, 15, 24, 26.

Dizziness: GV 4, 20, 21, 24; Bl 6, 8, 11, 62; GB 20; St 8, 36; Ht 5, 6; TW 23.

Epilepsy: GV 6, 8, 15, 16, 18, 19, 20, 22, 24, 26, 27; CV 12, 13, 15; GB 13, 15; Bl 3, 15, 63; Ki 1; Sp 4; Ht 7; SI 3, 8; C/P 5, 7, 8.

Meningitis: GV 4; Lu 11; Ki 1.

Stroke: GV 15, 20, 26; GB 15, 20, 26; GB 15; CV 8; Lu 5.

Heat stroke: GV 26; GB 20.

EMOTIONAL, MENTAL, AND BEHAVIORAL DISORDERS

Anger: St 6; Ki 8, 9; Bl 18.

Crying, excessive: Ht 7, 9; Ki 1; St 41; Sp 14; Lu 5; GB 24, 23; C/P 7.

Delirium: GV 12, 16, 26, 27; SI 5; St 39.

Depression: GV 18; Lu 3; Ht 1.

Fear/fearful nature: GV 16, 20; C/P 3, 5; Ht 7; St 36, 45; SI 7; Lu 10; GB 9.

  in child: TW 18.

Paranoia: Bl 66.

Foolishness: CV 15; Ht 7; Ki 4.

Forgetfulness: GV 11, 20; Bl 15, 38; Ki 7; Lu 7; Ht 3, 7.

Hallucinations: GV 16; Bl 12, 61.

Hysteria: GV 14, 26.

Insomnia: Ht 7; Lu 9; SI 1; Sp 1, 6, 9; Ki 3; Bl 13, 40.

Laughter excessive: Ht 7; Lu 9; SI 1; Sp 1, 6, 9; Ki 3; Bl 13, 40.

Lust: Sp 20.

Madness/insanity: GV 1, 6, 8, 18, 24, 26, 27; CV 14, 15; Bl 11, 12, 15, 57, 58, 62, 65; Ki 9, 20; GB 9, 12, 13, 36; St 24, 40, 41, 45; SI 3, 5, 7; LI 6, 7.

Sadness: Bl 4, 6, 8, 14, 37, 41, 67; GB 8, 12, 39; St 23, 36, 41; Lu 4, 10; TW 15; GV 8; Ht 8.

Nerves weakness: GV 20.

Sleep excessive: GV 22; Ki 1, 4, 6; Lv 1, 10; St 45; LI 12, 13; TW 8, 10.

To calm spirit: C/P 5; Ht 7; GB 20; GV 24.

Thinking excessive: Sp 5.

Worry: SI 7.

CHEST

Any problems: C/P 6.

Cancer: St 16, 18, 20.

Clavicle pain: St 12, 41; LI 1; Lu 9; Ki 24.

Diaphragm pain or cramp: Sp 17; CV 14; Bl 17.

Breathing difficult: Lu 1; LI 5; CV 14, 15; GB 10, 23; St 9.

Chest pain: CV 14; 18, 19; Ht 8; Ki 22, 27; TW 10; GB 10, 43; St 39.

Ribs pain: TW 6; Lv 14; GB 34; St 16; Bl 18; Ht 2.

Sternum pain: Bl 18; Lv 2, 3; CV 13, 14.

Esophagus:

   cancer: CV 17.

   spasm: CV 22; Lu 8; LI 2.

Breast:

   any problems: Bl 46.

   abscess: Lu 10.

   cancer: GB 21.

   inflamed: St 18; GB 21; Ki 24.

   lactation excessive: CV 8.

   lactation insufficient: St 8, 18; CV 17; C/P 1; SI 1, 2; Sp 12.

   pain: C/P 1; CV 19; St 34.

   swelling: St 36; Sp 18.

   tumor: CV 17; St 15; Ki 23.

RESPIRATORY

Lung cancer: Bl 38.

Congestion: CV 16; Ki 25.

Pleurisy: CV 18; Lu 1, 5; Bl 11, 12, 17, 19; St 12, 18, 40; Sp 1, 4, 10; Lv 13, 14; Ki 8.

Pneumonia: Bl 13; LI 13; Lu 1.

Tuberculosis: Lu 1, 5, 7; LI 10; GV 12, 13, 14; Bl 12, 13, 38, 40; St 36; GB 19; Ki 1, 27.

Asthma: CV 6, 17, 20, 22; GV 14; Bl 12; Lu 1; St 40; Lv 14.

Breathing problems: Ki 23, 27; GV 14; GB 21; St 20.

Bronchitis: CV 19, 22, 23; Bl 12, 13, 17; Ki 24, 25; Lu 3.

Coughing: GV 12, 14; CV 17, 19, 20, 21; Lu 5, 7, 9, 10, 11; SI 1, 2, 15; C/P 2; Bl 13, 14, 37, 60; GB 11; Sp 6, 18, 20; Ki 4, 22, 27.

Coughing blood: CV 15, 17, 18, 22; Lu 5, 6, 9, 10; LI 13; SI 15; C/P 3; Ht 7; Bl 13, 15, 18, 38; Ki, 2; Lu 2, 3; GB 42.

Emphysema: CV 17; St 16; GV 14; Lu 5, 8.

Hiccups: CV 22; St 18; Bl 17; TW 17; Ki 3; St 5.

Shortness of breath: CV 14; Bl 13; St 16; Lu 2, 5, 10.

Sneezing: GB 4; Lu 5; Bl 12.

Breathing stopped: Ki 1.

HEART

Attack: Ht 9; SI 1.

Diseases in general: GV 11.

Angina pectoris: C/P 3, 4, 6, 7, 9; Ht 4, 5, 6, 7, 9; CV 15; Ki 1; Lv 3; Sp 4; Bl 15.

Carditis: Lu 5.

Pain: C/P 2, 5; Ht 1, 3; Lu 4, 8, 9; CV 8, 14; GV 8; Lv 13, 14; Bl 16, 64; CV 17.

Palpitations: C/P 5; Ht 5, 6, 7, 9; CV 13, 15; Bl 15; Ki 1, 4; GB 19.

ABDOMEN

Any problems: C/P 6; CV 6.

Cramps:

upper: CV 14.

lower: CV 11; Bl 63; GB 25.

gas: CV 3, 7; St 29.

with swelling: CV 4, 6, 10, 12; Lv 13, 14; Ki 1; Sp 4, 5; St 36; Bl 44, 45, 48.

Hernia: GV 1; CV 3, 4, 14; Lv 1, 2, 3; Ki 1, 14; Sp 13; St 27, 36; Bl 55, 63; GB 40.

Pain: CV 10; Ki 5, 8, 17; Sp 12, 13; Bl 16, 29.

Peritonitis: CV 13; Lv 14; Bl 63.

DIGESTIVE PROBLEMS

Anorexia: CV 9, 12; GV 6, 20; Sp 4, 6, 8; St 13, 19, 20, 22, 36; Bl 17, 20, 22, 43, 64; Ki 17, 21, 27; GB 28; TW 10; Ht 8.

Appetite:

excessive: St 45; CV 3.

but remains thin: Bl 20, 25; Sp 7.

can't eat but likes to drink: Sp 20.

Emaciation: LI 15; Bl 21; CV 6, 10; GB 19.

Flatulence: Bl 21; Sp 7.

Indigestion: CV 13; Lv 13; Bl 21, 47, 48, 66; Sp 3, 5, 7, 9, 13, 16; Ki 20; GV 5.

STOMACH AND SPLEEN

Stomach:

   all problems: CV 8, 12; C/P 6; St 25, 36.

   ache: CV 10; GV 7; St 44; Sp 4; Bl 21.

   bleeding: CV 12; Bl 21.

   cancer: CV 12; Bl 17, 21; Sp 4.

   pain: CV 13, 15; Sp 2, 5; St 43; Bl 43; Ki 18.

Nausea: Lu 4; Ht 1.

Seasickness: C/P 5.

Vomiting: CV 10, 23; GV 14; Lv 13; Bl 6, 12, 13, 14, 17, 20, 22, 37, 41, 44, 61; Sp 3, 4, 5; St 36; Ki 3, 4, 6, 24, 25, 26; Lu 8; C/P 3, 5.

Dry heaves: C/P 5; Ht 4; Bl 19.

Morning sickness: C/P 5.

Spleen, all problems: Sp 4, 5, 6; Lv 13.

SMALL INTESTINE AND LARGE INTESTINE

Small intestine:

   all problems: CV 8; St 25, 36.

   inflammation (enteritis): Bl 17, 20, 27.

   pain: GV 4; Lv 1, 2; Sp 6; Bl 27; St 22, 30, 37.

Large intestine:

   all problems (incl. appendix and ileocecal): St 25, 36, 41; GV 1; CV 5; Bl 25, 26.

   dysentery: CV 4, 12; Bl 22, 27, 28, 29, 43; Lv 8; Ki 7, 21; St 25, 39; Sp 3.

   colitis: Bl 15, 17, 18, 19, 21, 22, 23, 25; LI 3, 4, 11; St 25, 36, 37, 44; Sp 3, 4, 6, 15; Lv 2, 3, 12; CV 6, 10, 12, 13, 14, 17; GB 20; C/P 6; Lu 9.

   rectal bleeding: GV 1; Lv 8; Bl 25, 51, 57.

   cramp: Bl 30.

   hemorrhoids: GV 4, 6; Bl 24, 27, 56, 58, 65.

   constipation: CV 6, 12; Lv 1, 2, 3, 13; GB 34; Ki 3, 4, 6, 7, 15, 16,

18; Sp 2, 5; St 3; Bl 27, 28, 30, 31, 32, 33, 34, 49, 56; St 57; TW 6.

diarrhea: GV 1, 4; CV 4, 8, 12; Lv 3, 13, 14; GB 25; Sp 1, 5, 9, 14; St 22, 36; Bl 26, 28, 30, 31, 32, 33, 34, 35, 41, 42, 43, 44, 65.

LIVER AND GALL BLADDER

Liver enlargement: Bl 18, 21, 23.

Gall bladder problems: Bl 19.

Hepatitis: Lv 13, 14; St 45.

Jaundice: GV 6, 16, 28; CV 9, 12, 13, 14; Bl 12, 15, 18, 19, 20, 21, 44; Sp 5; St 45; Ki 1; C/P 6, 8; Ht 7; SI 3, 4; LI 2.

KIDNEY AND BLADDER

All problems: Ki 3, 7, 27; Bl 23, 47, 64.

Kidney inflammation: Bl 22, 23, 25, 47; Ki 2, 3.

Kidney weakness: Bl 23, 29; GV 4.

Bladder problems: St 28; Lv 4; CV 2, 6, 7; Bl 28; Ki 10.

Blood in urine (hematuria): CV 3, 4, 6; Bl 23, 32, 43; Lu 9; LI 8.

Urinary incontinence: CV 2, 3, 4; Bl 23, 53; GV 3, 4; St 8; Lu 10; Sp 11; St 22.

REPRODUCTIVE SYSTEM

All problems: Ki 2, 3, 6, 7; Bl 22, 23, 24, 47; Sp 6, 10; St 29, 36; CV 26.

Impotence/no sex drive: CV 3, 4; GV 4; Bl 15, 23; Ki 10.

Sterility: CV 4; Bl 23; Lv 11; St 25, 29, 30.

Premature ejaculation: GV 3.

Prostate problems: CV 3, 4; Bl 23.

Menses:

amenorrhea (lack of flow): GV 2; Lv 3; CV 4; Ki 7; Bl 23; St 28, 29; Sp 6.

dysmenorrhea (painful and difficult): CV 3, 4, 6; Bl 23; Sp 6, 10; Ki 1, 4.

excessive/metrorrhagia (bleeding between periods): CV 2, 3, 7; Lv 1, 2, 3; GV 4; Ht 5; Sp 1, 10; St 30; Bl 31, 32, 33, 34, 55.

Ovaries inflamed: St 27, 29, 30; Bl 31.

Uterus:

cramp: Ki 1, 4.

hemorrhage: Sp 2; Lv 1, 2; CV 2, 5, 6; Sp 1, 6.

inflammation: CV 2; C/P 6; Ht 7; Sp 6, 10; Bl 28, 30, 31, 32, 33, 34; St 30, 33; Ki 3; GB 26.

Vagina:

discharge: CV 4, 7; Ki 12; Lv 5.

inflammation: Sp 9.

itching (pruritus): Ki 2, 6; CV 3, 7; Ht 8; Lv 8.

pain: CV 1, 3; Lv 1, 14; St 29; Bl 23, 55.

spasm: Ki 6.

swelling: CV 1.

PREGNANCY

Any problems during: GV 20.

Miscarriage: CV 8.

Morning sickness: CV 5.

Breech: Bl 60, 67; Sp 6; Lv 14; GB 21; St 30.

Postpartum bleeding: Sp 6; Lv 3.

Lactation: See CHEST: Breast.

Note: During pregnancy, never apply strong pressure to the teeth and gums or to these points: CV 4, 5, 11; Lv 14; Sp 2, 6; St 25; Bl 60, 67; GB 21.

SKIN

Any problems: Bl 13, 17, 54; LI 4, 11; Sp 10.

Acne: Lu 2; LI 11.

Itching: Bl 13, 17; LI 4, 11; TW 6; St 32.

Perspiration:

absent: TW 15; St 39.

excessive: Ht 6; SI 3; TW 10; Bl 17; GB 38; Ki 2, 8; Sp 14.

MUSCLES

Cramps: GV 4; Ht 4; Bl 8, 63; Ki 1; Lu 5; C/P 5; SI 5; TW 18; Sp 2.

Spasms, twitching: Bl 53, 65.

BONES

Cancer: Sp 5.

Joint pain: Bl 58; GB 38; Sp 2, 3, 5.

Broken bones: Do points on area broken on opposite side, with general treatment; Ki 1.

NECK

Cramps: GV 13, 14; Bl 10; GB 20, 21; LI 14; SI 8, 9, 10; extra points on neck.

BACK

Any problems: Release bladder meridian and Shu points; Bl 40; Ki 1, 10; GV meridian. Back problems are yin problems.

GENERAL SYMPTOMS

Addictions: St 8, 15, 25, 40; CV 10, 14; GV 20; GB 20, 34; Ki 1; Sp 1, 6; C/P 7; Ht 7; Lu 7; TW 6; LI 4, 11; SI 3.

Coldness: Ht 2; St 22; Bl 45; Ki 3, GB 7.

Diabetes: Bl 13, 17, 18, 20, 21, 23; St 33, 36; Sp 6; CV 4; GV 4; Ki 2, 3, 5, 7; LI 4, 12; Lv 1, 2; extra point between diaphragm and liver Shu points (marked as glucose point in Shu point chart).

Edema/water retention: CV 3, 7, 8, 9, 12; Sp 4, 6, 8, 9; Ki 7, 8; Bl 20, 23, 28, 39; GB 28; St 25, 28, 36, 43, 44; St 45; GV 4; Lu 7; LI 4, 6.

Fatigue: TW 8; St 36; Bl 18, 20; Ki 2; Lv 2, 3, 4, 14; CV 12.

Fever: Bl 11, 12, 53, 54; GV 4, 14, 16; LI 4, 6, 11; Sp 3; Lu 15.

Hay fever: Bl 2; LI 4, 19, 20; Lu 1, 9; GB 20; St 36, 18; GV 16, 20, 23.

Headache: See HEAD.

Hiccups: See RESPIRATORY.

Heat stroke: See BRAIN.

Hypertension: C/P 8, 9; Sp 1, 6; St 36.

Influenza: GV 13, 14; GB 20; Lv 14, 11; Lu 1, 9; Ki 3; Bl 22.

Insect bites: LI 11; Sp 10; Bl 54.

Laziness: Sp 5; St 40; Bl 43.

Mucus excess: St 40; LI 4, 11; Lu 1, 9.

Paralysis: GB 30, 31, 34, 39; LI 8, 9, 11, 15; Lu 7; GV 20; St 8; Bl 15; points in the area of paralysis.

Meningitis: See BRAIN.

Stroke: See BRAIN.

Parkinson's disease: Ht 3; St 33; CV and GV meridians.

Shaking of body: Bl 57, 58, 63; GB 38.

Sleep problems: See BRAIN.

Shock: GV 26, 27, 28; Ki 1; Bl 7, 42, 61, 63; LI 19.

Smoking, to stop: CV 20; GV 24; Ht 7; C/P 6; Lu 4, 7; LI 4, 13; St 36, 40; Sp 8.

Snoring: GB 2, 20, 40; GV 26; Bl 15, 18; SI 19; CV 12.

Tapeworm: St 25.

Tetanus: Ki 2.

Tuberculosis: Bl 13; St 36, 40; Lu 5.

Vomiting or motion sickness: See STOMACH AND SPLEEN.

Weakness: Bl 23, 38; CV 3, 4; St 36; Ki 1.

ENDOCRINE POINTS

Pituitary: GV 16, 18, 20; Ki 11; Bl 52, 60; GB 5, 37; LI 10, 15, 16, 19; Sp 5, 6.

Thyroid:

hyper: St 9, 10; CV 15, 23; Bl 15; GV 14, 15, 20, 23; Ht 7; Lv 2; LI 4, 6, 13, 19.

hypo: GV 14, 20; Lu 9, 10; Ki 7; TW 3; LI 4, 6, 13, 19.

Parathyroid:

hyper: Bl 11, 58; GB 30; St 36.

hypo: SI 3; C/P 6; Lv 2, 3; CV 15.

Thymus: Sp 2; Bl 11; GB 34; CV 17, 18.

Adrenals:

hyper: Sp 6; C/P 7; Bl 47.

hypo: Ki 7; Bl 47; Sp 6; GV 11, 16, 18.

Cortisone deficiency: GV 16; Sp 2, 6; Bl 18, 20.

Testicles:

hyper: St 30; CV 3, 4; Bl 60.

hypo: Ki 11; GV 3, 4, 5; Bl 47.

Ovaries:

hyper: Ki 2, 13; Lv 3; Sp 6; CV 4.

hypo: Ki 7, 13; Bl 67; GB 37; Sp 6.

Arthritis:

general: LI 4, 10, 11, 12, 15; St 36; Sp 4; TW 6; GB 20, 21, 30, 34, 39; GV 14.

specific: general points above plus points in the affected area; Parathyroid points; Adrenal hypo points.

Dietary note: Arthritis is from excessive yin and yang. Eat lots of vegetables, grains (especially millet and kasha in winter, corn in summer), and sea vegetables; stay away from acidic foods, hot spices, drugs, coffee, commercial teas, sugar, and excess meat and salt. Get exercise, breathe well, and chew well. Do not hold in feces or urine.

Index